PATAÑJALI AND ĀYURVEDIC YOGA

AUTHOR'S OTHER PUBLICATIONS*

1. Yogasūtras of Patañjali: A Scientific Exposition, Clarion Books, New Delhi
2. Yoga for Integral Health, Hind Pocket Books, New Delhi
3. Ayurveda: A Way of Life, MLBD, Delhi
4. Ayurveda for Life: Nutrition, Sexual Energy and Healing, MLBD, Delhi
5. Stress-free Work with Yoga and Ayurveda, New Age Books, New Delhi
6. The Kamasutra for Women, Penguin-India, New Delhi
7. Ayurvedic Food Culture and Recipes, Penguin-India

* These books are also published in various European languages, and also in English in America and in Hindi in India. *The Kamasutra for Women* is also published in Malyalam.

Cover design by the author: Śṛī Amarnāth ice liṅgaṁ representing Śiva, the symbol of the universe and *Kāleśvara,* the God of time (photograph taken by the author on 17th July, 2000). The cosmos is called *brahmāṇḍ* in Sanskrit which literally means an egg of immensity and human being in this immensity is *kṣudra brahmāṇḍ* which means small egg of immensity; or *vyasti* - the fragmentary universe. Significance of egg is void. Void is *śūnya,* i.e. nothing, zero (*bindu*), the world seed and the source of all energy. *Bīja* or seed signifies the continuum through propagation. The universe arises from the void and dissolves into the void and the wheel of eternal time goes on turning.
(Cited from author's television lecture in Germany - *Man and the Cosmos in Hindu Tradition,* 1990)

Patañjali
and
Āyurvedic Yoga

(A comparison of classical yoga with Āyurveda; the practice of Āyurvedic yoga in our daily lives for healing, maintaining health and harmony)

VINOD VERMA

MOTILAL BANARSIDASS PUBLISHERS
PRIVATE LIMITED • DELHI

First Indian Edition: Delhi, 2001

ISBN: 81-208-1826-1

Also available at:

MOTILAL BANARSIDASS

8 Mahalaxmi Chamber, 22 Bhulabhai Desai Road, Mumbai 400 026
236, 9th Main III Block, Jayanagar, Bangalore 560 011
41 U.A. Bungalow Road, Jawahar Nagar, Delhi 110 007
120 Royapettah High Road, Mylapore, Chennai 600 004
Sanas Plaza, 1302 Baji Rao Road, Pune 411 002
8 Camac Street, Kolkata 700 017
Ashok Rajpath, Patna 800 004
Chowk, Varanasi 221 001

Printed in India
BY JAINENDRA PRAKASH JAIN AT SHRI JAINENDRA PRESS,
A-45 NARAINA, PHASE-I, NEW DELHI 110 028
AND PUBLISHED BY NARENDRA PRAKASH JAIN FOR
MOTILAL BANARSIDASS PUBLISHERS PRIVATE LIMITED,
BUNGALOW ROAD, DELHI 110 007

Dedication

This book is dedicated to my spiritual guru, Patañjali, to my Āyurvedic guru, Āchārya Priya Vrat Sharma and to all other great sages of yoga and Āyurveda who provided us with this wisdom beyond space and time.

Foreword

Āyurveda deals with life in wide perspective and prescribes and guides the way of life which is conducive to happiness and ultimately leads to bliss. In the definition of Āyurveda (*Caraka-Saṃhitā, Sūtrasthāna,* I, 41) '*tasya hitāhitam*' means that it describes what is wholesome and unwholesome causing equilibrium and disequilibrium respectively in body and mind. Equilibrium is health and disequilibrium is disease (*Caraka-Saṃhitā, Sūtrasthāna,* IX, 4). Technically, '*hita*' may be taken as '*sama yoga*' while '*ahita*' as *viṣama yoga. Yoga* in the sense of application or use is of four types—*atiyoga, ayoga, mithyā yoga* and *sama yoga.* Out of these, the first three are the cause of misery while *sama yoga* leads to happiness but is very difficult (*sudurlabha*). '*Yoga*', in general, denotes *sama yoga* which is also indicated by the word '*yukti*' (proper application). The management of health and disease with judicious application of diet and drug is termed as '*yuktivyapāśrayā* (based on yukti). The same idea is conveyed by '*yogobhavati duḥkhahā*' in the *Bhagavadgītā.*

Somatic diseases are caused by imbalance of *vāta, pitta* and *kapha* while mental disorders take place by *rajas* and *tamas.* Āyurveda does not categorise *sattva* with *rajas* and *tamas* as has been done in the other systems. From the Āyurvedic point of view, *sattva* is perfect and pure, it is achieved with yogic methods and it leads to bliss. It is also sometimes known as '*śuddha sattva*'. In this respect, Āyurveda also differs from the *Bhagavadgītā* that places *sattva* along with *rajas* and *tamas* (collectively *triguṇa*) and describes the superman as *triguṇātita* (while in Āyurveda it is *dvidoṣātita*). Scholars while trying to correlate these may think that in *triguṇa, sattva* is tinged with *rajas* while *śuddha sattva* has no trace thereof.

Body, including mind, carries on by equilibrium of *dhātus* (*samayogavāhni*) and gets diseased by their disequilibrium. *Samatva* (equilibrium) is *yoga* which brings efficiency and activity in body and mind (*karmasu kauśalam*) and also alleviates all miseries (*duḥkhasaṃyogaviyoga*).

In Āyurveda, *yoga* (the union of mind and spirit by meditation) and *mokṣa* (liberation) are similar to those in Patañjali. In *yoga* and *mokṣa,* there is cessation of all sensations, the latter having complete cessation while the former leading to it (*Caraka-Saṃhitā, Śarirasthāna,* I, 137-139). *'Ātmasthe manasi sthire'* denotes the stage of *samādhi.*

Prajñāparādha (intellectual error) is the root cause of almost all disorders. It is due to error in any of *dhī* (knowledge), *dhṛti* (restraint) and *smṛti* (recollection). When all of them are functioning normally, the person stays like *sthitaprajña* and is free from disorders. Mental disorders are treated with these three (*jñana-vijñana, dhairya, smṛti)* supported by *Samādhi* (*Caraka-Saṃhitā, Sūtrasthāna,* I, 58).

As one of the three types of therapies, '*sattvāvajaya*' (control of mind) is described by Caraka. It is defined as controlling mind from unwholesome objects (*Caraka-Saṃhitā, Sūtrasthāna,* II, 54). This definition becomes complete when the above factors like *jñana-vijñana* etc. are included therein. In fact, author's newly coined term 'Ayurvedic yoga' is nothing but '*sattvāvajaya*' in all its aspects.

Patañjali is a recognised authority equally in *Yoga,* grammar (*vyākaraṇa*) and Āyurveda and the author of the *Yogasūtra, Mahābhāṣya* and redaction of *Caraka-Saṃhitā* (see introductory verses in *Cakrakapāṇidatta's* commentary on *Caraka-Saṃhitā*).

Thus, it is interesting and informative to compare the views of Patañjali on *Yoga* vis-a-vis those in Āyurveda.

Dr. Vinod Verma is a prolific writer who has written a number of books on health based upon traditional Indian therapeutics. Particularly, she has been devoted to *yoga* and has contributed a lot on its theoretical and practical aspects with Patañjali as her inspiring spirit. Now in the present work, she has tried to demonstrate how Patañjali's Yoga put in practice as Āyurvedic yoga can transform life and divinise body and mind. I congratulate Dr. Verma for this novel approach in the field of *yoga* and medicine which would revolutionise the approach to management of health and disease.

Varanasi **PRIYA VRAT SHARMA**
May 7, 2001

Contents

Note to the Reader

The yogic exercises, postures, breathing practices and other health-care suggestions provided in this book are for educational and self-help purpose and are not intended to replace the services of a physician. No medical claims will be accepted in this direction.

To use the herbal or yogic methods provided in this book for commercial purpose, the agreement and permission from the author are required. Those who violate so will be subjected to jurisdiction.

Note to the Reader

Preface

Both, yoga and Āyurveda are primarily concerned with the body. In the Indian tradition, the word 'body' is used for the totality of our physical being. What kindles life in the body is soul, which is only energy without any material substance or qualities and is eternal. Thus, soul is the cause of consciousness. Body is ephemeral and is the seat of all pains and pleasures. It is the medium of all our experiences, feelings, learning, sufferings and joys. We enjoy food, sex and other sensuous pleasures at diverse levels. We suffer when we are sick or our bodily energy dwindles or we lose someone we love or incur a financial loss. As long as we live, we love, we accumulate, and we feel very involved with the world as well as with our physical self. But one day, we have to leave all this behind because the soul departs from the body and we no more remain the embodied self. The seers in India tried to seek immortality through the methods of yoga, which involved recognising our real and eternal self, the soul and its oneness with the eternal universal energy. To achieve this aim, a person has to conquer the senses through the control of mind and reach the spiritual level, that is, consciousness in its purest form. On the one hand, senses and mind are constantly attracted to the fascinating universe, but on the other hand, the senses are controlled through the power of mind. To achieve spiritual level, one has to have good health conditions, otherwise it is not possible to be uninvolved with the body. For example, a person with a stiff body, or blocked nose or heaviness in abdomen may have difficulty even to sit still continuously for a certain period of time to obtain a thought-free mind.

Āyurveda, the science of life of ancient India, is primarily concerned with optimum quality of life, longevity and freedom from ailments. It teaches us that for a healthy, disease-free life and for obtaining maximum vitality and energy, one has to attain equilibrium at physical, mental and spiritual levels. Since Āyurveda is a science, it concerns with the physical, mental and social health as well as environment and not with the religious and philosophical beliefs and values of people or the ultimate spiritual goal of the terrestrial existence.

To obtain mental and physical harmony is essential in both Āyurveda and yoga. For example, negative qualities like excessive attachment, desire, greed, anger, jealousy should be avoided because they lead to ill health. In yoga, for getting rid of the ego to attain the realisation of one's real self, soul (spiritual lucidity), it is essential to get rid of these negative traits. The following citation from the Āyurvedic text of Caraka (6th century BC) illustrates the basic similarities between the two disciplines:

> **'Allurement is the greatest cause of misery and its renunciation eliminates all miseries. As a silkworm brings forth threads leading to its own end, the ignorant and greedy person creates allurement from the sense objects. One who is wise enough to identify the fire-like sense objects and readily withdraws from them is not attracted by misery due to the absence of initiation and conjunction.'**[1]

Although yogic practices existed in India since eternity, yoga became a separate school of thought after the great sage Patañjali wrote a systematic treatise on it, known as the Yogasūtra. The text is in four Parts with a total of 195 aphorisms or sūtras. It is the first systematic text on yoga and was written around 6th century BC, the time which is also considered to be the golden period of Āyurveda. Patañjali's exposition of yoga is an explicit analysis of the working of human mind as well as experience of various layers and dimensions of human consciousness. The author expounds the ways to achieve the limitless human capabilities and powers. The way to self-exploration is through human body, which is of primary importance to attain the spiritual goal. At the same time, the body is also the seat of sensuous pleasures and emotional fulfilment. It experiences all worldly sorrows and joys. For enhancing pleasure, increasing one's work capability and creativity, facing life with courage, for strength and stability and to experience the intensity of being alive, we need to explore the unlimited power of human mind just the same way as for experiencing the deeper dimensions of consciousness. Yoga teaches to control the thought process, to stop the chain of thoughts and to achieve stillness of mind to awaken the dormant human energy. Whether we use this

[1] *Caraka Saṃhitā, Śarīrasthānam,* I, 95-97

energy for the worldly pleasures or spiritual is up to us. Yoga teaches the techniques of liberation from the cyclic physical existence and to achieve immortality. Āyurveda tells us to lead a harmonious, disease-free life with enhanced vitality and vigour. However, the fundamentals of both yoga and Āyurveda are based upon *Sāṃkhya*, one of the six major schools of thought of ancient India. The aim is different in yoga and Āyurveda but the medium for both these disciplines is the body.

The purpose of this book is to comprehend the concept of body in both these disciplines. The second aim is to develop new, simple methods from this ancient wisdom in order to achieve health, peace and harmony in our lives. An average human being does not aspire to be a yogi but the first few steps of yoga, which are also recommended by Āyurvedic sages can enrich human life and can provide techniques to gain energy. Spiritual lucidity can help us tremendously in everyday situations, like managing crisis and maintaining inner discipline. Is it important to have inner discipline for good health, for improving the quality of life and for warding off ailments? Yes, indeed it is! Lack of self-discipline sows seeds of many ailments. Learning to bend the mind according to time and situation, not feel dissatisfied and accept with smile what comes in one's way and have strength and courage to go through ups and downs of life are the results of inner discipline. These qualities provide a solid ground for good physical and mental health.

In our times, most people seem to be racing with time and this is particularly true about the urban population. There is too much *rajas* or activity which leads to imbalance. If there is no balance between *sattva* (stillness, harmony, and peace), *rajas* (activities and movements) and *tamas* (inactivity and rest of the senses and mind), we are no more in tune with the cosmos. The inner human organisation rebels, becomes disorganised and there are disorders at diverse levels. In ancient Indian mythology, there is often mention of gods and demons and the war between the two. The gods are *deva* and demons are *asura*. *Deva* in Sanskrit means divine, shining, celestial, god. *Asura* means, that which is not in harmony. The word *sura* means rhythm and *asura* is that which is arrhythmic. Both *deva* and *asura* have human bodies but in their description *asura* are pictured as those with unnatural activities like eating excessively, killing and paining others, roaming around at night and sleeping during the day and disturbing nature by interfering in its organised system.

Present day human beings have developed many *āsurī pravṛttis* or imbalanced essential nature, which give rise to many disorders, ailments and diseases. Such activities seem comfortable and enjoyable at the present moment but lead to disastrous results. The purpose of this book is to invoke the awareness of what is *āsurī* within us and to work towards developing *sattva* that will lead to equilibrium, harmony and peace. All this can be done by modifying our thinking process and by using simple methods to do so.

I have divided this book into five Sections. The Section I provides an introduction to the ancient Indian tradition and yoga and Āyurveda in its historical, philosophical and cultural perspective. The Section II is on the *Yogasūtra of Patañjali* and the essence of the yogic wisdom with the view of using techniques described by Patañjali in our daily lives. The Section III provides in brief, the fundamentals of Āyurveda with its principles and practice in daily life. The Section IV is on the integration of yoga and Āyurveda, their similarities and differences. The fifth and last Section is on Āyurvedic yoga and its practice in our daily lives. This Section has five Chapters and these contain thirteen different programmes for the practice of, what I call 'The Āyurvedic yoga'. Some of these programmes do not require any extra time and involve only diverting your mind when you are doing your usual activities.

The latest developments in science and technology and rapid modes of communication have changed our lives extensively. We should effectively take advantage of the new techniques and should not lose our balance with the changing pace of life. I see myself and other writers and researchers like me as medium to bring the wisdom of ancient sages stylised for our modern way of living. I would welcome comments and experiences of the reader.

Note for this English Edition for India

I write in English and normally my books are published in the US and are also translated and published into different European languages as well as in Hindi without making significant changes. But this book has a slightly different history. I translated and commented on the Yogasūtra of Patañjali in 1986-87. Patañjali's immense source of wisdom became a never-ending task for me. Finally, the book was published in 1996 in English. Later, for the German edition, I added to this book another 100 pages on Āyurvedic yoga and this was published in 1998. For this present English edition, I have summed up the essence of Patañjali's sūtras and the Āyurvedic yoga is appearing for the first time in English for Indian market. Those interested in the details of the Yogasūtra, their translation, glossary etc. may refer to my other book as well.[2]

The present book is more of a practical guide for using principles of yoga and Āyurveda in day to day life, specifically in our modern times when people generally say, 'I do not have time'. In fact, one does not need to have free time for many of the things mentioned in this volume. It is more the mental attitude that needs to be changed. Two thousand six hundred years ago, our great sage Caraka said that the root cause of many ailments is *asantoṣa* (dissatisfaction). With the hectic pace of life and an ever-increasing race with time, we are losing our age-old traditional values especially in the urbanised sections of our society. I suggest that there is a mid-way and that we do not have to be technologically primitive in order to continue our lives with the invaluable source of wisdom from our past. Our rich heritage is beyond space and time and that is why Patañjali is translated at least in fifty different versions in English and in numerous other languages of the world. Āyurvedic wisdom is also spreading all over the world very rapidly. I feel pained when I see some foreign companies selling us Āyurvedic formulations under the name of herbal medicine.

I request my country people to value our infinite treasures for their well-being and health. We are at a path of rapid economic progress and let us join hands to make it a mental and spiritual progress as well. It is a saying that when Lakṣmī, (the goddess of wealth) comes alone without Sarasvatī, the (goddess of wisdom), she is riding on a crow and brings destruction along with wealth. Let us not get dazzled with our newly acquired technology and integrate *sattva* in our lives and society. Let us all make an

[2] Verma, V. *The Yogasūtra of Patañjali: A Scientific Exposition*, 1996, Clarion Books, New Delhi.

effort to continue the tradition of the rishis to make our lives peaceful and pleasant . Let us open our minds with tolerance and love and spread the message of our *sattvic* tradition throughout the world.

January 2000

VINOD VERMA
The New Way Health Organization. NOW.
A-130, Sector 26, Noida 201301, Uttar Pradesh

Acknowledgements

First of all, I am grateful to my publisher Motilal Banarsidass for making the Indian edition of this book possible. Mr. Rajeev Prakash Jain was very convincing about the importance of the English-speaking public in India. Though the American English editions of my books are distributed in India but the value of dollar being very high, they were not as easy to access as my Hindi editions. It is very important for me that I am read in my own country and can contribute a little in continuing our great ancient traditions.

I am grateful to all my friends and family for adjusting to my crazy schedules and helping me in all possible ways. Seema and Rajesh Vikram Emerson who were my next door neighbours while I was writing this book helped me in all odds. Rajesh has taken all those photographs where I appear. My nephew Abhinav modeled for some of the yoga pictures and my nieces Gayatri and Shruti also did their participation. My special gratitude is to my friend Heinrich (Dr. Heinrich Heyne) to give me courage and assistance at every step and for getting computer equipments and solving other associated problems.

I am grateful to the National Museum, New Delhi for providing me the picture of The *Mahāyogī* (Figure 1).

Pronunciation Note

In this book, the Sanskrit words are transcribed in Latin alphabet according to the international transcription codes. Given below are the details of transcription and sound equivalents in some Eupopean languages, wherever possible to facilitate the Sanskrit pronunciation.

VOWELS

अ	or	अ	a	Short	as in 'above'. For example, the word 'Yoga' is pronounced without a long 'a' at the end and is roughly 'yog'
आ	or	आ	ā	long	as in 'army', 'calm', etc. It is like the vowel 'a' in French and Italian
इ			i	short	as in 'illustrate', 'illusion', etc.
ई			ī	long	as in 'machine'
उ			u	short	as in 'bull'
ऊ			ū	long	as in 'rule'
ए			e	short	as in 'prey' or 'é" in French
ऐ			ai	long	as in 'bain' in French
ओ			o	short	as in 'go'
औ			au	long	as in 'cow'

CONSONANTS

Guttural

क	ka	as in 'colour'
ख	kha	as in 'khaki'
ग	ga	as in 'guide'
घ	gha	
ङ	ṅa	nasal

Palatal

च	ca	as in 'China'
छ	cha	
ज	ja	as in 'jam'
झ	jha	
ञ	ña	a little as 'singen' in German

Cerebral

ट	ṭa	as in 'true'
ठ	ṭha	
ड	ḍa	as in 'drum'
ढ	ḍha	
ण or रा	ṇa	

Dental

त	ta	as in French and Italian
थ	tha	stronger than as in 'thunder'
द	da	as 'd' in French
ध	dha	
न	na	as in 'number'

Labial

प	pa	as in 'pump'
फ	pha	as in 'pharaohs' or 'shepherd'
ब	ba	as in 'banana'
भ	bha	
म	ma	as in 'machine'

Sibilant

श	śa	as in 'shred'

ष	ṣa	as in 'sure'
स	sa	as in 'sweet'

Diverse

य	ya	as in 'yellow'
र	ra	as in 'run'
ल	la	as in 'lavender'
व	va	as in 'vacuum'

Aspirate

ह	ha	as in 'hundred' or 'heruber' in German

Mixed Consonants

ऋ	ṛ	pronounced as in 'rich'
क्ष	kṣa	pronounced as in 'ksha'
त्र	tra	
ज्ञ	jña	pronounced between 'jya' and 'gya' with a nasal sound

Signs

	ṃ	nasal
	ḥ	as in 'hallo'

Sign 'ऽ' (*avagraha*) represents the sound of 'अ' with a pause.

Sign (*halanta*) is below a consonant (म्, न्) and makes it short sounding

Happiness and misery arise due to the contact of the soul, sense organs, mind and sense objects. When the mind is withdrawn from the senses and is concentrated on the soul, it identifies itself with the soul and a supernatural power comes forth.

***Caraka Saṃhitā, Śarīrasthānam*, I, 138-139**

Avidyā or ignorance is considering the non-eternal, the impure, the distressful and that which is not soul, to be eternal, pure, joyful and soul.

***Patañjali, Yogasūtra*, II, 5**

SECTION I

Ancient Indian Tradition and Yoga and Āyurveda in their Historical, Social and Cultural Perspective

The historical data from the West or our historians with the western domination say that our culture began from the Indus Valley civilisation which dates back to 3000 BC and that this culture was invaded by the so-called Āryans who came, perhaps, from central Europe. According to this tentative information, Āryans must have plundered the existing civilisation with well planned and well organised cities and established themselves in India. Perhaps a thousand years later, Āryans wrote the brilliant books of wisdom, the four major Vedas.

Indian scholars and some other well-known indologists do not agree to this theory of our past. Somehow, it does not seem very rational to think that a great civilisation like that of the Indus, where extremely well planned cities were built and there was a very well organised society, was so easily plundered and destroyed by the invaders. The Indus Valley civilisation, which was spread in the vast Northwest areas of the subcontinent was so easily brought to ashes or pushed back to the southern part of the subcontinent, seems very unlikely. This civilisation must have been at its peak, as there were established trade links with other major civilisations like Mesopotamia and Babylon. It does not seem rational to think that the nomadic Āryans became so brilliant in a short span of time to give to the world the great languages, timeless wisdom of the Vedas and other bodies of ancient Indian literature.

There must have been integration and enrichment by diverse people from diverse parts of the world, which gave rise to culture and profound philosophical and religious traditions on the subcontinent. It is difficult to ascertain the antiquity of this tradition, which continues until today. In the context of yoga, a seal of Mohen jo Daro depicts a yogī-like figure sitting in *padamāsana* (lotus posture). Some scholars call it prototype of Lord Śiva. Different animals surround the *Mahāyogī* or the great yogī and that strengthens this belief, as one of the names of Lord Śiva is *Paśupatinātha*, the protector of animals (Figure 1).

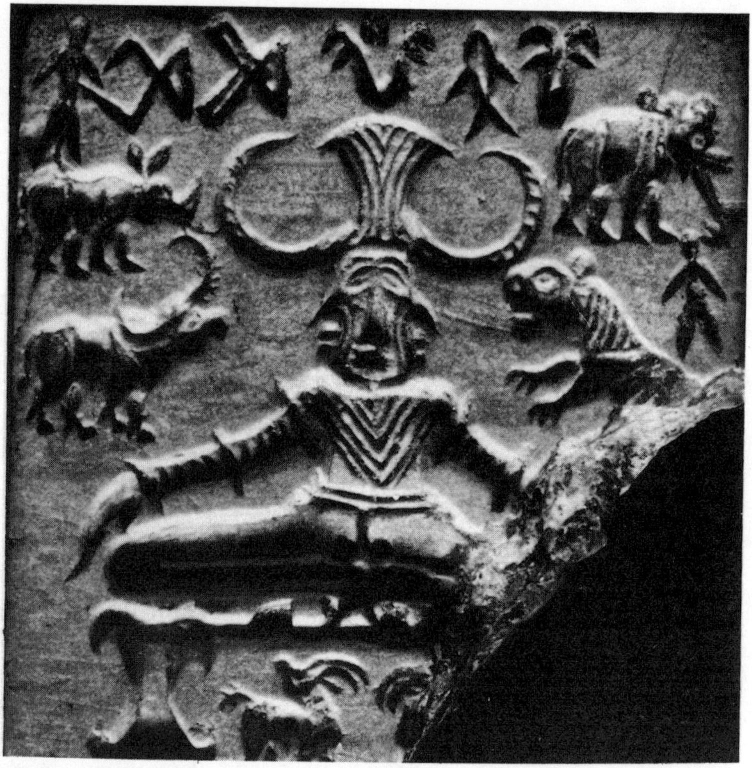

Figure 1. The *Mahāyogī* (the great yogī), prototype of Lord Śiva, on a Mohen jo Daro seal of Indus valley civilisation, 3000 BC.

The Indus Valley civilisation, as it is called, developed along the river Indus or Sindhu. The neighbouring Persians could not pronounce 'S' and, they said Hindu instead. From Persia, the word Hindu was communicated to the rest of the world and the people of the subcontinent became known as the Hindus in the rest of the world, further giving rise to the words like Indu, Indus, Industhan, Hindusthan and so on. Whatever we may call them, the people of the subcontinent developed a great wisdom for life and cosmic theories of the universe. They wrote about cosmogony, cosmology, existence itself and the oneness of all cosmic phenomena.

The *Vedas, Brāhmaṇas* and *Upaniṣads* were written and the life was lived according to certain principles. These principles were in fact the imitation of the natural phenomena and human actions were in harmony with the cosmic principles. It was believed that human existence was a smaller system, which belonged to and was similar to the bigger cosmic system on a smaller scale.

Sanātana dharma

The principles for life based upon the cosmic principles were called *sanātana dharma* by the ancient Indians. *Sanātana dharma* is not a religion but a Weltanschauung. As already mentioned above, it does not only talk of the human beings and the cosmos but also of the cosmogony. It is continuity in time and it denotes the Eternal norm or the cosmic system in cyclic order. The essence of the teachings of *sanātana dharma* is that *Brahman* or the Universal Soul pervades all in cosmos and is the cause of life. All what exists is cyclic. Even the phenomenal world is cyclic. That is why a wheel called *dharmacakra* or the cosmic wheel (Figure 2) represents *sanātana dharma.* The cosmic wheel revolves around its immutable axis, *Brahman* or the Universal Energy. The

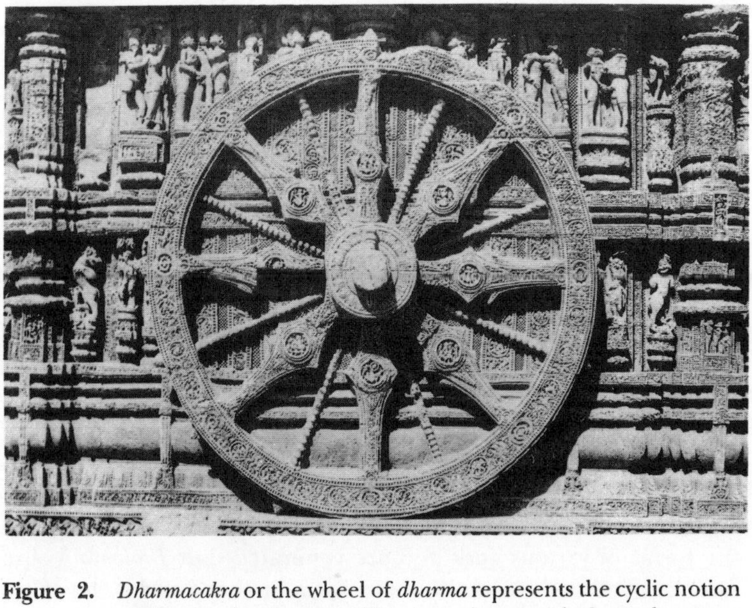

Figure 2. *Dharmacakra* or the wheel of *dharma* represents the cyclic notion of time and existence. This is a photograph from the stone chariot of Sun god from the Sun Temple of Konārk, Orissa.

wheel in our national flag also represents the *dharmacakra*. *Dharma* denotes the order governing the cosmos in all its manifestations, cosmic, religious, social etc. Different doctrines were developed on the Indian continent for a common goal and they all are part of the *dharma*.

It is important to know that there is nothing as 'Hinduism' as this vast tradition of the Hindus is not bound by certain sets of rules and regulations to be followed and the followers are not required to pray to or believe in certain God or god-like figure and so on. It has no founder or no special norms. It is technically wrong to use the word 'Hinduism' and in fact, *dharma* cannot be translated as religion. From the description that follows, it will be clear that the Hindu *dharma* is far from being a religion. It is a cosmic system where human beings are also there. There is no God who can be responsible for the good or evil of the world. It is the *karma* of each one of us which is responsible for our pains and pleasures. Each individual is responsible for his or her good or bad luck. It is a vast and well-organised system that works with cause, effect and substratum. A human being cannot assign his/her goods or evils to a particular god. Each individual accumulates his or her *karma* and these unfold themselves at the appropriate time and situation. There is a cycle of life and death and the quality of the next life depends upon the previous *karma* of an individual. The only way to get rid of this cycle is through yoga. Similarly, there is bigger cycle of the phenomenal world and its dissolution. Time is eternal and hence neither the individual nor the world comes to an end and therefore a *cakra* or wheel represents *dharma*. This idea will be clearer after the description of the other concepts and of *Sāṃkhya* thought which is the basis of yogic and Āyurvedic philosophy.

Brahman or the Universal Soul

One may describe *Brahman* as the cosmic energy or the Universal soul that puts life into all things and is the cause of all that exists. It is not a God. There are many gods in the Hindu tradition. The cosmic entities like the sun, moon, rivers, mountains etc. acquire the forms of various gods and are venerated. But *Brahman* is the essence of all and it is without any form or shape and is the cause of being. In the ancient literature, it is addressed simply with a pronoun 'that'. In *Muṇḍaka Upaniṣad,* it is described as follows:

> **'That which cannot be seen, nor seized, which has no origin, which has no properties, which has neither ears nor eyes, which has neither hands nor feet, which is eternal, diversely manifested, all-pervading, extremely subtle and imperishable, the wise regard it as source of all beings, all creation.'**[1]

Before proceeding further, I would like to point out two things here.

1. Western mind or the westernised Indians often become confused with the numerous gods and the multiple philosophies of the Hindu tradition. There are many gods, yet there is no God. It is merely the energy which pervades all and which is the cause of life. The answer to this is that the various manifestations of nature are given the form of gods. Gods have symbolically philosophical significance and I have explained that towards the end of this Section. Besides that, the gods are stepping stones to reach the unembodied *Brahman.* They make the path easier for us, the embodied.
2. Unfortunately, some western scholars look at history and tradition of ancient India in the form of compartmentalisation.[2] In fact, that is their way of looking also at their own history with the idea of rise and fall of the empires and beginning of new eras, like the fall of Roman empire and the beginning of the Christian Era. Whether it is the East or the West, we cannot dichotomise events, time and happenings. These scholars try to separate the tradition of the Vedas from so-called Hinduism. They try to build the strict boarder lines between the doctrines and beliefs, which evolved in the Indus Valley and the planes of the Gaṅgā. It is important to understand that a constant evolution and blending of the ideas, beliefs, rituals and customs took place in the Indian sub-continent in the past. It was not a replacement of old tradition and doctrines with the new ones. Until today, in the traditional Hindu ceremonies and

---

[1] *Muṇḍaka Upaniṣad,* I, 6.

[2] Michelle George, 1977, *The Hindu Temple,* Harper and Row, New York, pp.15-17. A.L. Basham, 1971, *The Wonder that was India,* Fontana Books, Calcutta, p. 354.

in the daily prayers of temples, the Vedas and Upaniṣads are recited. Historian A. L. Basham has also emphasised this fact as follows:

'The *Ṛg Veda* and the great body of oral and religious literature which followed it in the first half of the first millennium BC belong to the living Hindu tradition. The *Vedic* hymns are still recited at the weddings and funerals and at the daily devotion of the *Brahman*.'[3]

According to *Ṛg Veda*, the universe was built (not created) by Viśvakarmā. In fact, god Viśvakarmā is still worshipped in India as the maker of the universe (Figure 3). On Viśvakarmā day, which falls a day after the Divali festival, people worship the implements of their trades and professions. Divali festival falls on the new moon at the end of October or beginning of November and traditionally denotes the end of the financial year. On this day, the goddess of wealth and well-being, Lakṣmī, is worshipped. Thus, worshipping tools and implements marks the beginning of the new financial year. In some other parts of India, god Viśvakarmā is worshipped four times a year during the change of seasons as the architect and the creator god.

A question is raised about Viśvakarmā as a builder and how he built this universe. The answer is found in *Mahānārāyaṇa Upaniṣad* as follows:

'The something in which all things assemble and disperse,
on which the gods have their seats,
is That, the imperishable, the supreme firmament...
That something with which space
and heaven and earth were filled,
by whose means the sun warms,
by whose means the water generates life,
is That, order and truth,
the supreme *Brahman* of the sages?
Navel of the universe,
That sustains all things'[4]

---

3 A. L. Basham, Ibid, p. 31.

4 *Mahānārāyaṇa Upaniṣad*, I, 3-5.

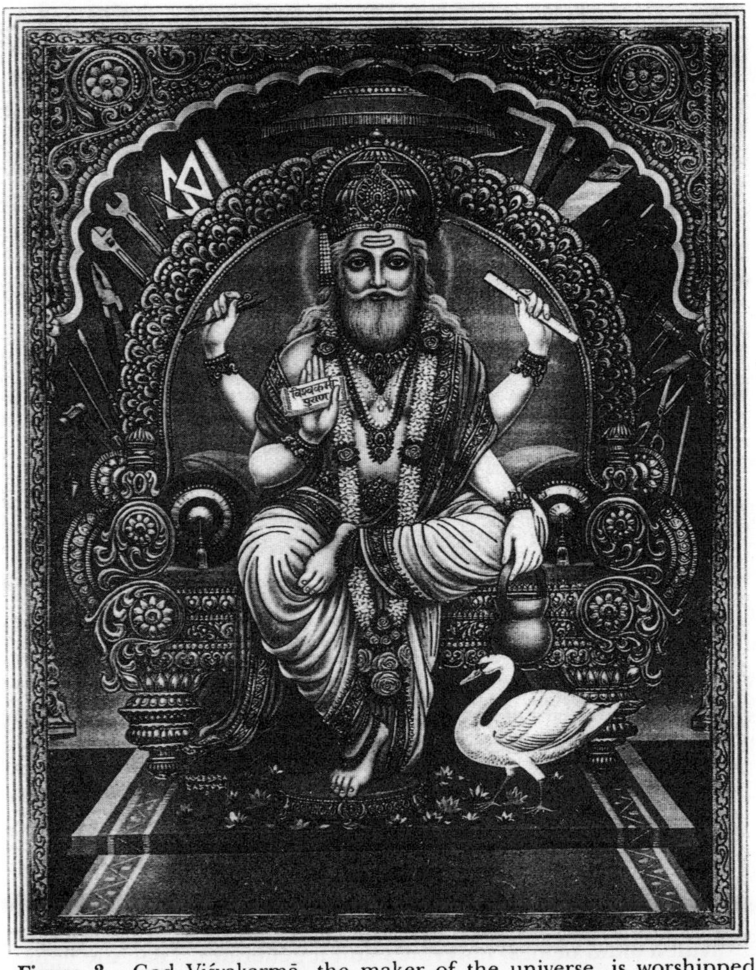

Figure 3. God Viśvakarmā, the maker of the universe, is worshipped along with the implements of one's trade. It is to show the gratitude to the builder of the universe for providing them the means of livelihood and also to show the gratitude to the implements of one's trade, which are the means of earning livelihood.

Brahman is the essence of all life, it is the cause of the phenomenal world and existence. In *Chāndogya Upaniṣad,* Uddālaka teaches about the universal reality to his son Śvetaketu as follows:

> **'Fetch me a fruit of the Banyan tree.'**
> **'Here is one, Sir.'**
> **'Break it.'**
> **'I have broken it, Sir.'**
> **'What do you see?'**
> **'Very tiny seeds, Sir.'**
> **'Break one seed.'**
> **'I have broken it, Sir.'**
> **'Now what do you see?'**
> **'Nothing, Sir.'**
> **'My son, Said the father, what you do not perceive is the essence, and in that essence, the mighty Banyan tree exists. Believe me my son, in that essence is the self of all that is. That is the truth and that is the self and you are that self Śvetaketu!'**[5]

The period of *Vedas, Brāhmaṇas* and *Upaniṣads* is termed as the *Vedic* period. Later, in the *Bhagavad Gītā,* this spiritual message was conveyed in the form of devotional songs. But the fundamental *Vedic* thought about the universal reality remained the same in this body of literature.

> **'Supreme Eternal *Brahman,* which can be called neither being nor non-being... without any senses, unattached, supporting everything, free from qualities and enjoying qualities, ...within all beings, immovable and also movable, by reason of its subtlety, imperceptible, at hand and far away is That. Not divided amid beings, it devours and it generates. That, the light of all lights is said to be beyond darkness, wisdom, object of wisdom, by wisdom to be reached, seated in the hearts of all.'**[6]

In the *Bhagavad Gītā,* Kṛṣṇa is teaching Arjuna about *dharma, Brahman, yoga, karma* and so on in eighteen discourses. Kṛṣṇa is the representation of *Brahman* (Universal Soul) and Arjuna represents a human and they are popularly known as *Nara* (Arjuna) and

[5] *Chāndogya Upaniṣad,* VI, 13
[6] *Bhagavad Gītā,* XIII, 12, 14-17.

Nārāyaṇa (Kṛṣṇa). The relationship of a human being to the Universal Soul and *dharma* is expressed as follows in the *Bhagavad Gītā*:

> **'Arjuna, those who have no faith in *dharma* fail to reach Me and revolve in the path of world of death. The whole of this Universe is permeated by me as unmanifest Divinity, and all beings rest on the idea within Me. Therefore, really speaking, I am not present in them. Nor all those beings abide in me; they behold the wonderful power of My divine Yoga. Though the sustainer and creator of beings, in reality, I do not dwell in those beings.'**[7]

It is important to understand that *Brahman* is the principal, and we, as well as our perceptual reality are its manifestations. *Brahman* is all-pervasive energy and therefore it cannot be expressed in the form of single, personified God. Numerous Hindu gods symbolically represent its different manifestations. The philosophical symbolism of the gods along with their pictures is given later in this Section.

There is a cosmic oneness and the unmanifest *Brahman* permeates all that exists and that is why for the Hindus, anything can be the object of veneration, a river, a tree, a stone, a mountain, the sun, the moon, stars, a mantra, another human being or a guru and so on. The Hindu tradition is not theistic. *Brahman* is unembodied and it is difficult for the embodied to reach the unembodied. The gods provide the stepping stones and make this path easier. For a better comprehension of the Eternal energy, in *Ṛg Veda*, it is compared to the human form.

> **'A thousand are the heads of a man-cosmos,**
> **a thousand his eyes and thousand his feet!....**
> **He is all that is, all that was, all that will be....**
> **From his mind, originated the moon,**
> **from his eyes, the sun,**
> **from his mouth the fire, and**
> **from his prāṇa, the air came forth.**
> **From his navel originated the space,**
> **And from his head, the heaven;**
> **the earth originated from his feet,**
> **and directions (east, west etc.) came from his ears.'**[8]

---

7 *Bhagavad Gītā,* IX, 3-5.

8 *Ṛg Veda,* X-90, 1, 2, 13, 14.

When we go through the *Vedic* scriptures, we find that the sages persisted again and again that *Brahman* should be confused neither with gods and nor should It be visualised in the form of some personification. In *Mahānārāyaṇa Upaniṣad*, *Brahman* is described as follows:

> **'That in which all things assemble and disperse,**
> **on which the gods have their seats,**
> **is That the imperishable, the supreme firmament....**
> **That with which space, heaven and earth were filled,**
> **By whose means the sun warms,**
> **by whose means the waters generate life,**
> **is That order and Truth,**
> **the supreme *Brahman* of the sages?**
> **navel of the universe, that sustains all things...**[9]

In *Kena Upaniṣad*, the same idea is expressed in different words:

> **'That which speech cannot express but**
> **through which speech is expressed....,**
> **That which thought cannot conceive but**
> **through which thought is thought....**
> **That which sight cannot see but**
> **through which sight sees....**
> **That which hearing cannot hear but**
> **through which hearing is heard....**
> **That which breath cannot breathe but**
> **through which breathing is breathed....**
> **That, indeed is the immensity and**
> **not what is here worshipped.'**[10]

As this Section of the book will proceed, these concepts will be clearer. To understand the base of the *Sanātana dharma* and the Hindu tradition, it is important to understand the concept of *karma.*

Karma

According to the Hindu tradition, the cosmos is a well-organised and dynamic whole, where there is a constant change and trans-

[9] *Mahānārāyaṇa Upaniṣad,* I, 3-5.
[10] *Kena Upaniṣad,* I, 4-8

formation. There is nothing without a definite function and there is exact selection of means for the realisation of a definite end. Nothing happens without reason or fortuitously. Nothing is wasted; everything is transformed from one state to another; there is no finality. Time is transformation from one state to another and that makes us perceive one moment different from another.

Human beings represent the cosmos in its microform. The soul in the human body is a part of the Universal Soul or *Brahman*, which is eternal and is the cause of being. The material reality of the world as well as the human body is made of five elements, which are ether, air, fire, water and earth. After death, the five elements the body is constituted of go back to their cosmic pool. The soul or the essence of being of an individual is the human continuity. It is bound to the cycle of birth and death, called *saṃsāra*, due to *karma* or deeds. *Karma* are the inherent nature of our existence. These are the deeds we perform during the time we are alive. Deeds of one life are responsible for the quality of the next life. The variations in the appearance, nature and behaviour of the human beings are due to sum total of the impressions of their past *karma* called *saṃskāra*. It is through our intellect and power of discretion that we are supposed to discriminate between good and bad *karma*. By doing good *karma*, one can also alter the effect of past bad *karma* or vice versa. Although one has to account for one's past *karma*, it does not mean that all is pre-determined during the life of an individual. The human freedom lies in the performance of the present *karma*, which is entirely dependent upon an individual's discretion and will.

The *karma* theory is erroneously understood by some as deterministic and is used to shirk off their responsibilities. In fact, it is quite the other way round. If we are suffering, it is because we have sown the seeds for it and we are reaping the harvest. We have the freedom to make best out of this situation with our discretion and will. We have a chance to learn a lesson from this situation and with determination, we can perform better deeds for altering the present to some extent and for improving our future. *Karma* theory inspires us for devotion to our duty and to perform the virtuous acts of compassion, kindness and sacrifice. Some of the virtuous deeds which accumulate good *karma* are to give alms, to help the poor and the needy, to donate our services for the society, to help in pious acts like education, to save the environment from degradation, to participate in greening of the earth and to take part in any other cause for the well-being of humanity and our planet. Good deeds should not be done with a mercenary attitude. One should indulge in these activities selflessly without wanting anything in return. Good *karma* is a powerful protector against the sufferings of this world. It generates courage and provides spiritual strength. With these two, one acquires the sense of discretion and is guided and protected by it.

The *karma* with its cause, effect and substratum give rise to a self-governing system. We make our own path as we go ahead in life. Human effort has a supreme value. Misdeeds are punished, if not in this life, then in the next. A convict may escape the court punishments by having false witnesses, but the escape is not possible in the ultimate court of the bigger system based upon the cause and effect of *karma.* Then the only choice left is to lessen the effect of the past bad *karma* with further good *karma* and meditation.

In Indian society, the theory of *karma* is very deep-rooted. This gives people courage to accept their miseries with facility. This is also the reason that donations are a very important part of this culture. From the poorest to the rich, *karma* constitutes a part of the daily conversation. People may not be afraid of the gods when they are trying to cheat or do some other such deed, but being reminded of *karma,* many refrain from such acts. When someone narrowly escapes an accident or any other disaster, it is often said that some past good *karma* came to rescue.

Saṃsāra

We see that the inherent nature of our existence is the performance of *karma*...and this binds us to the cyclic time. We are born to die and die to be reborn. This cyclic human journey is called *saṃsāra.* This is how the whole cosmic system is organised and it is perfected to function on its own. Then why sages wanted liberation from this cycle? Why they thought that *saṃsāra* was painful? We come in this world and we love, possess, own, learn, build, create and so on. One day we have to leave all what we have accumulated and learnt and all those we love and that too without any prior notification. When we are reborn again, we have to redo everything again. What a pain!

Human brain has its limitations. It is capable of storing memories only for one life as it is destroyed with death. The remains of *karma* called *saṃskāra* drive us to the next body. Once the next body is there, they further unfold in terms of our aptitudes, personality, interests and so on. In a way *saṃskāra* are subtle forms of memory on a large scale of time. But because of the limitation of our memory, which is limited to one life, it becomes difficult to grasp concepts, which are on a larger scale of time than one life.

It is perhaps easy to grasp the idea of pain from *saṃsāra,* if we take time on a smaller scale. Imagine yourself being called in a room again and again and then each time you are told to leave after a period of few minutes. This happens hundred times a day. It is an awful experience as you go in just to leave and as soon as you leave, you are waiting to be called inside. It is very irritating and painful experience. You will never like to be in the same situation again. If you have this kind of job, you will make every effort to find some alternative work, which is more peaceful. It is nearly the same situation when we have to undergo the cycle of birth and death. It is even worse as we forget all our learning too and have to relearn from A B C... again. Thus, the sages in ancient India sought and found ways to achieve eternal freedom from the cycle of birth and death.

Mokṣa or liberation from the cycle of birth and death (*saṃsāra*)

According to the Hindu tradition, the ultimate aim of life is to seek liberation from the mortal world and to submerge one's individual eternal self (the soul) into *Brahman* or the Absolute. This state of submersion into the eternal energy is called mokṣa.

The soul, which is the cause of being in the body, is not involved with the *karma* an individual does. It is like a reflecting glass that reflects the activities of the mind. However, an individual soul is loaded with *saṃskāra* (the results of the remains of sum total of the *karma*) at the time of death. It is like a computer disc, it has on it whatever you put on it. There are many *karmic* accounts to be settled with so many individuals, places and situations when a human being dies. Compelled by this force, the individual soul acquires a new body and is reborn. It undergoes an unending cycle of birth and death. Liberation from this cycle is possible only through yogic methods by dissolving the effect of *karma* through meditation. When the effect of *karma* is finished, the individual soul is liberated from the bondage with the body and becomes a part of the Eternal Energy, *Brahman* or the Universal Soul or the Absolute. This bondage with the body is severed by the efforts of the adept of yoga and when this task is completed, the yogī is liberated while he is still alive. Yoga means oneness, dissolution or assimilation of two things. Thus, the eternal individual energy is assimilated into the great Universal Energy and the individual is liberated from the cycle of birth and death (See Figure 4).

Six orthodox schools of thought of Ancient India

To give a rational interpretation to the concept of *Brahman*, there originated many schools of speculative thought in the Hindu tradition. The doctrines, which followed the fundamental concepts of the Vedas, were termed as orthodox and other doctrines or religions, which did not accept the authority of the Vedas were termed as unorthodox (like the Jainism and the Buddhism). The six principal orthodox schools of thought of ancient India are: 1. *Nyāya*; 2. *Vaiśeṣika*; 3. *Sāṃkhya*; 4. *Yoga*; 5. *Mīmāṃsā*; and 6. *Vedānta*.

In all these different schools, the methods to achieve the aim may be different, but the goal is the same; that is to get rid of the cycle of birth and death and achieve the eternal freedom. In the present context, the two most important of these schools are *Sāṃkhya* and *Yoga*. *Sāṃkhya* provides the metaphysical basis for *Yoga* and the fundamentals of Āyurveda are also derived from *Sāṃkhya*. It is considered to be the oldest school of thought that has also influenced other doctrines including Buddhism.

The oneness of *Sāṃkhya* and *Yoga* is described in the *Bhagavad Gītā* as follows:

> **'In this world, two courses of spiritual discipline have been enunciated by me, O Sinless One! In the case of *Sāṃkhyas*, it proceeds along the path of knowledge, whereas in the case of *karma* yogīs, it proceeds along the path of action.'**

> **'Ignorant, not sages, speak of *Sāṃkhya* and *Yoga* as different but the same state is reached by the adept of both these disciplines.'[11]**

---

[11] *Bhagavad Gītā*, III, 3 and V, 4.

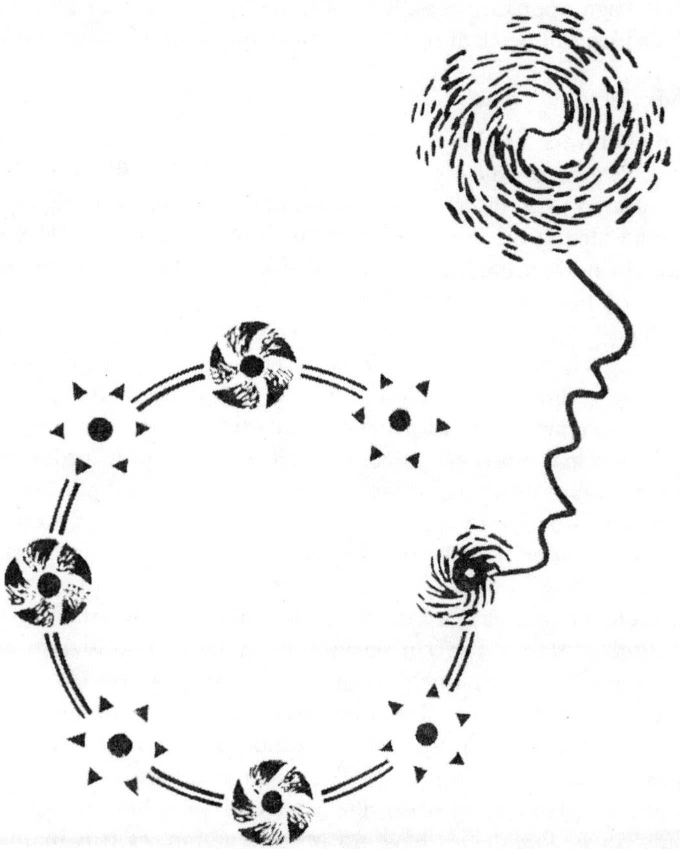

Figure 4. A figurative representation of the cycle of birth and death, *saṃsāra* and liberation from it. The soul loaded with *karma* enters from one body to another and the cycle of life and death (*saṃsāra*) goes on. Through yogic methods, an individual seeks liberation of the soul by dissolving *karma* and attaining oneness of the soul with the Universal Soul, *Puruṣa*

In fact, *Sāṃkhya* is a system of knowledge about the cosmos and Yoga opens up a path for the realisation of that knowledge. This idea will be clearer after the description of *Sāṃkhya* and Yoga.

Sāṃkhya

The founder of the School of *Sāṃkhya* was Sage Kapila and in the *Bhagavad Gītā* his name is mentioned (X, 26). The Sage is venerated until today on the island of Sāgara in the Gaṅgā's delta near Calcutta on the first day of the Hindu month of *Māgha* that falls in mid-January. It is believed that Sage Kapila spent the last part of his life on this island.

The term *Saṃkhyā* literally means number or count. This name is probably used because *Sāṃkhya* enumerates the principles of cosmic evolution by rational analysis based upon the principles of conservation, transformation and dissipation of energy. The phenomenal universe is considered as a dynamic order where there is an exact selection of means for the acquisition of a definite end. There is never a random combination of events and there is order, regulation, system and division of function.

According to *Sāṃkhya*, the phenomenal world begins when two principal energies combine with each other. These are *Puruṣa* and *Prakṛti*. *Puruṣa* is the Universal Soul; it has no substance and it does not have any qualities or *guṇa*. *Prakṛti* or the Cosmic Substance is the seat of all manifestations in the phenomenal world and has three qualities. But it cannot react on its own without *Puruṣa* that puts life into it. The *nirguṇa Puruṣa* (Universal Soul without qualities) also cannot act alone as it has no vehicle or substance. *Prakṛti* can have no urge to action, as it is inanimate. Thus, the phenomenal world begins only when these two energies fuse with each other. One gives life to another and the other provides vehicle to this unmanifest energy and the existence begins. *Puruṣa* is the Soul of the Universe and animating and living principle of *Prakṛti*. It is that which breathes life into matter and is the cause of consciousness. That is what is known as *Brahman* in the *Vedic* literature.

Before we proceed further, let us see what are the qualities or *guṇas* of *Prakṛti*. The three *guṇas* are *sattva, rajas* and *tamas*. *Sattva* is the quality of truth, virtue, beauty and equilibrium. *Rajas* is the quality of force and impetus which imparts motion. All that is energetic and forceful falls in this category. *Tamas* is the quality that restrains, obstructs and resists motion.

Before the formation of the phenomenal world, that is, before *Puruṣa* and *Prakṛti* come together, the three *guṇas* are in a state of perfect balance and the change in this balance is the cause of all phenomena. This balance is constantly changed through *karma,* which is the inherent nature of the combination of *Puruṣa* and *Prakṛti.* According to *Sāṃkhya,* salvation lies in realising the difference between the two ultimate realities of the universe through knowledge.

Let us see now various elements that originate with the combination of *Puruṣa* and *Prakṛti.* When these two cosmic principles combine with each other, *mahat* or the cosmic intellect originates. *Mahat* signifies the capacity to expand, reveal and ascertain. *Mahat* gives rise to the fourth component of *Sāṃkhya,* which is *ahaṃkāra* or the individuating principle. The fifth component is *manas* or the cosmic mind. These last three components or stages are not marked out in time but arise simultaneously. All these further give rise to five subtle elements or *tanmātra,* which are sound, touch, appearance, flavour and odour. From the subtle elements, the corresponding material or fundamental elements, the *mahābhūta* arise. In other words, the material world, made of five *mahābhūta* becomes a reality with intellect, identity of the self and power of thinking through the medium of five subtle elements (sound, touch, appearance, taste and odour). Let me put this in simple words for a better comprehension: 'with the sense of discretion or intellect, 'I' am able to think and realise through five subtle elements, the phenomenal world made of five *mahābhūta*'. It is becuase of the individuating principle or *ahaṃkāra* that one is able to become a perceiver of the existence. The perception of the reality of the phenomenal world according to *Sāṃkhya* is illustrated in Table 1.

Further evolution of the five subtle elements and the five fundamental elements is into five sense organs and five organs of action. The sense organs are the capacity to hear, feel, see, taste and smell. The five organs of action are to express, grasp, move, excrete and procreate. These ten-fold sense powers could have no existence without the corresponding subtle elements. For example, the power to hear would have no meaning without sound. The senses operate on co-related fundamental elements. For example, ether is the vehicle for sound for the power of

Table 1. Perception of the phenomenal world according to *Sāṃkhya* School of thought (the first three steps).

Puruṣa and *Prakṛti*	⇨	Intellect, Individuating Principle and Mind
Puruṣa and *Prakṛti* *Intellect, Individuating Principle* and *Mind*	⇨	Sound, Touch, Appearance, Flavour and Odour
Puruṣa and *Prakṛti* *Intellect, Individuating Principle* and *Mind* *Sound, Touch, Appearance, Flavour* and *Odour*	⇨	Perception of the reality made of five fundamental elements or *Mahābhūta* which are: Ether, Air, Fire, Water and Earth

hearing and light is the vehicle for perceiving the colours and forms of the universe through sense of sight and so on. The cosmic view according to *Sāṃkhya* has been illustrated in Table 2.

It is important to understand the relationship of five subtle and five fundamental elements. The five fundamental elements are in the order of their heaviness and complexity. Ether is related only to sound whereas in air there are both sound and touch. In fire, in addition to sound and touch, there is appearance. In water, there are sound, touch, appearance and taste. All the five subtle elements are related to the last fundamental element, the earth. This idea is illustrated in Table 3.

According to *Sāṃkhya*, time is eternal. Everything in the cosmos is cyclic and so is the formation of the phenomenal world. When *Puruṣa* and *Prakṛti* combine, there is the beginning of the phenomenal world and when they come apart, there is dissolution of the phenomenal world. This cycle goes on forever. Figure 5 shows a diagrammatic representation of the cosmic cycle with eternal time.

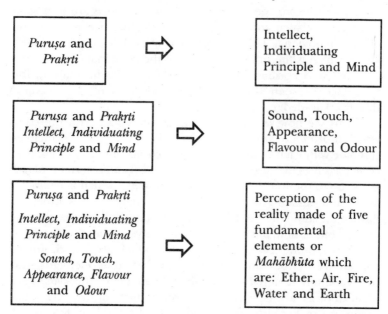

Table 2. An illustration of the evolution of various elements of cosmos according to *Sāṃkhya*.

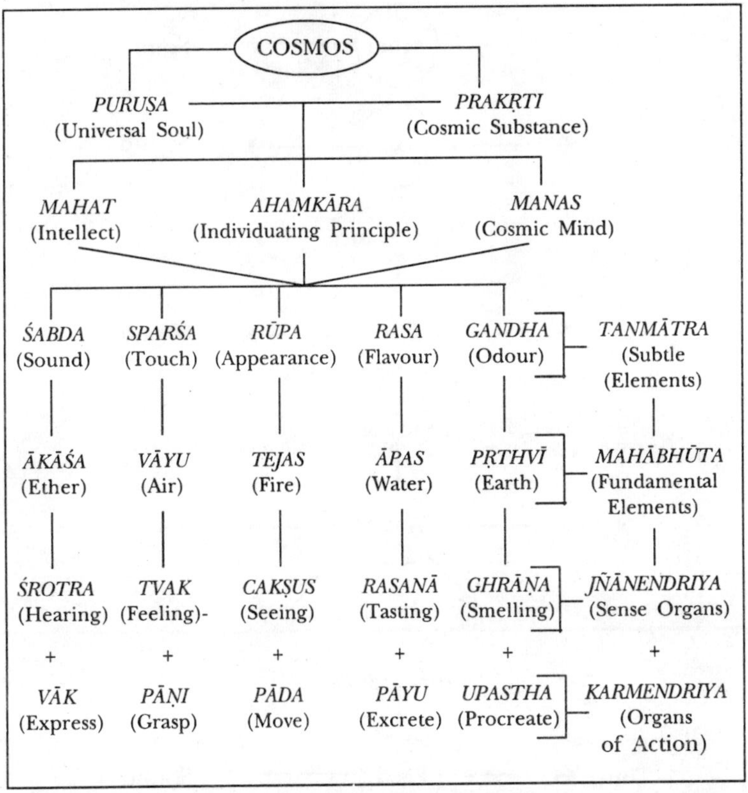

With the linear notion of time in mind, modern scientists believe in the theory that the universe came into being with a big bang fourteen thousand million years ago and one day its dissolution will take place with a big crunch. In the present context, with the cyclic notion of time, we may say that a small portion of a big circle gives a false impression of its being a line. In other words, the linear notion of time is the perception of only a part of the cosmic reality and not its entirety.

Patañjali's yoga

Sāṃkhya unfolds to us the knowledge about the cosmos and tells us that the salvation lies in realising the ultimate Truth. Following

Table 3. The relationship of subtle and fundamental elements.

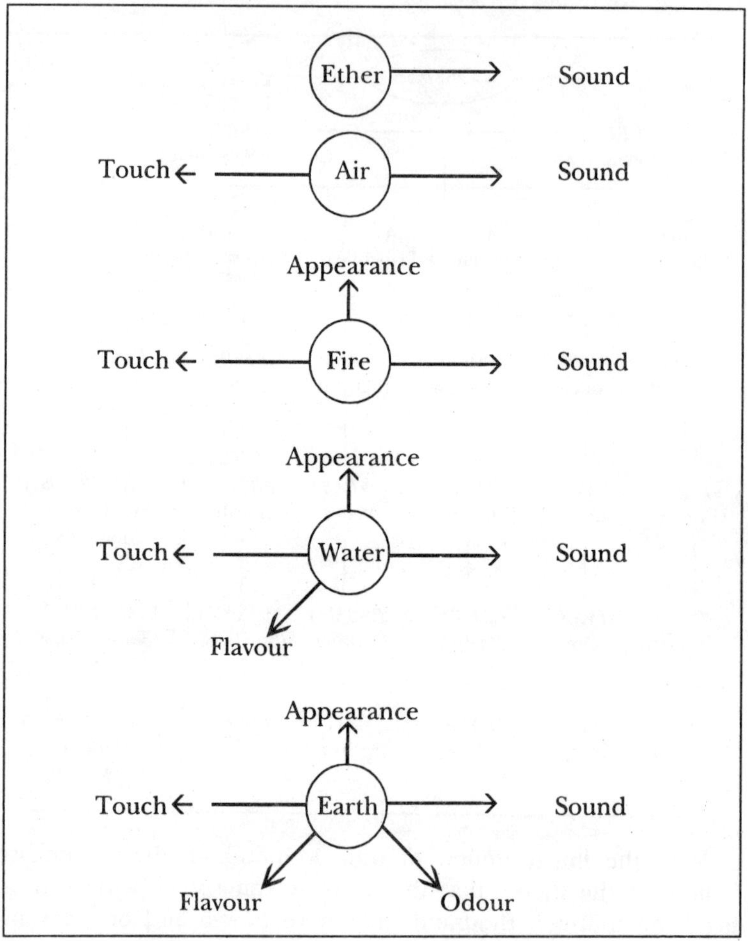

the path of *Sāṃkhya*, yoga gives the adept instructions and teaches the techniques for achieving the ultimate goal of attaining freedom from the cycle of birth and death and attaining eternity.

According to Patañjali, the soul, which is a part of *Puruṣa* is the real self of an individual. The nature of the soul is eternal whereas the physical self is time bound and ephemeral. To take one's physical self as the real self is ignorance or *avidyā*. Due to *karma*, the soul undergoes a cycle of life and death or *saṃsāra*.

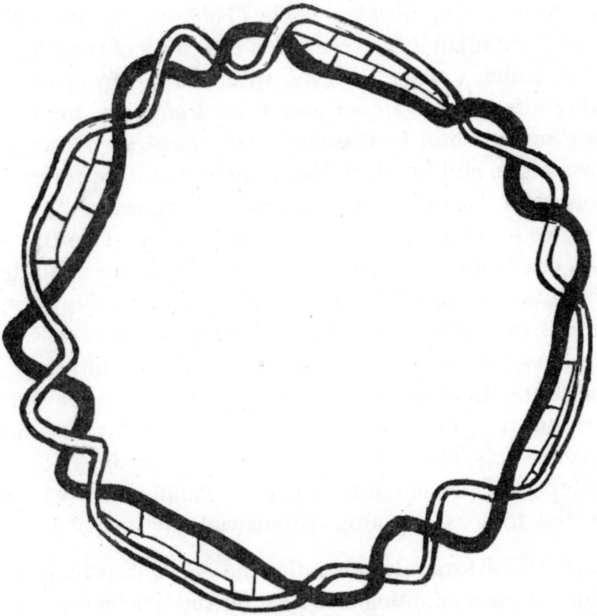

Figure 5. The cosmic cycle showing the eternity of time. *Puruṣa* and *Prakṛti* are together and there is phenomenal world. *Puruṣa* and *Prakṛti* are apart and there is dissolution of the phenomenal world.

The salvation from *saṃsāra* is achieved by recognising that the ultimate reality of one's being is soul and separating it from the involvement with the phenomenal world through the body. This is achieved through various concentration practices and by attaining mastery over one's senses. The soul is bound to the previous *karma* and the adept of yoga has to achieve the dissolution of these through various meditative practices. After having achieved that, the adept continues the meditative practices until the state of *viveka* or the discriminative knowledge is achieved. At this stage, the soul is dissociated from the body and is in the state of isolation or *kaivalya.* In other words, the soul of an individual becomes one with its ultimate cause, the Universal Soul or *Puruṣa.* Thus, the adept gains eternity and freedom form the cycle of birth and death. This state is also called *mokṣa* in other systems of *Vedic* thought as I have described earlier in this Section, and it is called *nirvāṇa* by the Buddha.

If we look at the *Sāṃkhya* Table (Table 2), we do realise that the yoga of Patañjali is the reversal of the cause of the phenomenal world. Patañjali's yoga involves withdrawing from the senses, achieving the pure state of *mahat* or *buddhi* by hindering the thinking process and by dissolution of *ahaṃkāra* or the individuating principle, and finally to bring the soul in its own pure nature, uninvolved in *Prakṛti* or the Cosmic Substance.

Thus, we see that the yoga of Patañjali is based on the atheistic *Sāṃkhya* doctorine. The greatness of Patañjali lies in understanding the human mind, its capabilities and in showing us the techniques to explore them through human effort. His scientific analysis of various levels of human consciousness and the methods to experience them can help us to explore our inner capabilities and profound levels of existence and the reality beyond that.

Unfortunately, some Western[12] as well as Indian scholars[13] have not understood the scientific aspect of Patañjali's work and have categorised him as adopting 'superficial theism'.

> **'He (Patañjali) merely rehandles the *Sāṃkhya* philosophy in its broad outlines, adapting it to a rather superficial theism.... Yoga is theistic, since it postulates the existence of supreme God (Īśvara); ....according to *Sāṃkhya*, the only path to salvation is metaphysical knowledge. Yoga accords marked importance to techniques of meditation.'**[14]

If one interprets Sūtra 23 of Part I of Patañjali's Yogasūtra which says that a profound devotion to *Īśvara* helps attain meditation, one can be easily misled as one of the meanings of the word *Īśvara* is God. Patañjali has a very precise meaning of this word and the succeeding sūtras show that the *Īśvara* here is the *Puruṣa* of *Sāṃkhya* and *Brahman* of the Vedas as he denotes it with the symbol OṂ (Sūtra 27). Sūtras 28 and 29 further clarify this view, which say that it is OṂ's repetition and reflection on its meaning which destroy all obstacle in the way of meditation and bring about consciousness of the omnipresent. Patañjali makes the symbolic significance of the Absolute very clear and no-where does he

---

[12] Mircea Eliade, 1969, *Yoga, Immortality and Freedom*, Princeton University Press, Princeton, p. 7.

[13] S. Radhakrishanan, 1923, *Indian Philosophy*, Volume II, London, p. 344.

[14] Mircea Eliade, 1969, *Yoga, Immortality and Freedom*, Princeton University Press, Princeton, p. 7.

describe his '*Īśvara*' as the embodied creator God. There is further discussion of this subject in Section II.

Sāṃkhya, yoga and Buddhism

Siddhārtha, later known as the Buddha was a spiritual leader in North India of the sixth century BC. Two hundred years after the Buddha, Buddhism established itself as a religion. The message of the Buddha was spread in Asia through the efforts of the great Indian emperor, Aśoka who reigned between 269 and 212 BC.

Teachings of the Buddha before the advent of Buddhism and consequently before the formation of its various sects are very much influenced by *Sāṃkhya* and the techniques of yoga. One of the Buddha's teachers was sage Arada who was a *Sāṃkhya* scholar. In both *Sāṃkhya* and yoga, self-mortification is not suggested; rather a disciplined life is recommended by following the eight-fold yogic path. The Buddha talked of a middle way, which was quite similar to these concepts. The Buddha also taught the concept of *avidyā* along the similar lines as *Sāṃkhya* and yoga. Also similar is the teaching of the Buddha that says, 'All is unhappiness in this world' and thus liberation is sought. Despite all this, there is a principal difference between the teachings of *Sāṃkhya* and yoga and those of the Buddha. The goal laid by the Buddha was *nirvāṇa,* which literally means 'going out' or to extinguish as a flame does. Thus, *nirvāṇa* is to extinguish oneself through the destruction of all that is individual and enter into communion with the whole universe in order to become an integral part of the great purpose. By becoming one with all that is, has ever been and can ever be; the state of being is submerged into the limits of reality.

For the Buddha, there was only one universal reality, whereas for *Sāṃkhya* and yoga, the phenomenal world is caused by the combination of the two basic realities, *Puruṣa* and *Prakṛti.* In *Advaita Vedānta* of *Śaṃkara* also, only one basic reality is admitted. In my opinion, the concepts of *Sāṃkhya* and yoga are more logical as compared to *Vedānta* and Buddhism. The point of view of *Sāṃkhya* and yoga, which says that the soul is involved with the body made of five elements and through personal effort an individual can isolate it from its cause and free it from the bondage seems very scientific to me.

Āyurveda in the context of *Sāṃkhya* and Yoga

Let us briefly look at the fundamentals of Āyurveda in relation to *Sāṃkhya* and yoga. *Caraka Saṃhitā* was compiled by the great sage and physician Caraka and is one of the most important treatises on Āyurveda. It was written around the same period as the Yogasūtra. In *Caraka Saṃhitā,* there is a mention of all the elements of *Sāṃkhya* and their interpretation is done in reference to the human body. I will discuss this in detail in Section IV of the book. But the important point to mention here is that both *Sāṃkhya* and Āyurveda take atheistic and non-religious stand. Fundamentals of Āyurveda begin from five fundamental elements or *Mahabhūta* mentioned in *Sāṃkhya.* These five elements form the material reality of the universe that also includes human body. The body is a vital organism because of the presence of soul, which is a part of *Puruṣa.* Soul is the cause of consciousness in the body. The body and soul are held together with *prāṇa,* the cosmic energy that we take inside us with respiration. Thus, the soul and the *prāṇa* make the body made of five elements into a vital and living organism, which is a complete system by itself. In the living body, for the performance of all physical and mental functions, the five elements take the form of three principal energies generally known as humours, called *vāta, pitta* and *kapha.* The principle of health lies in keeping the three humours in equilibrium so that they can perform their respective functions and co-operate with each other. If they are not in equilibrium, the perfected system of the body is disturbed and there are ailments and malfunctions.

One of the great things about Āyurveda is that it lays a great emphasis on human constitution or *prakṛti,* which can be seen from an individual's appearance and behaviour. The constitution is also related to the personality of an individual. By nutrition and other simple external measures, not only one can attain physical well-being, also these methods are used to treat personality problems like anger, irritation, impulsive behaviour and so on.

The three energies or humours are constantly influenced by external factors like nutrition, time, place, situations, mental state and behaviour. Āyurveda provides us with the knowledge of all these factors and with the wisdom of leading life in a way that helps maintain the mental and physical equilibrium and provides energy, vigour and long life.

The ailments and diseases are caused when there is a lack of equilibrium and balance at mental or physical level (individual *karma*) or social level (collective *karma*). They are also the results of the past *karma*. Āyurveda teaches us the nature of such imbalances, how to avoid them, how to cure disorders, handle epidemics and restore individual as well as social health.

Āyurveda is a science of life and health has a very extended meaning in this discipline. It teaches us to live in tune with the cosmic forces of which we are an integral part and also heal ourselves with natural remedies. The three types of disorders—innate, exogenous and psychic are interrelated and interdependent. For treating ailments and disorders, three-dimensional therapy—rational, mental and spiritual, is recommended simultaneously.

Like the rest of the Hindu tradition, this system of well-being does not believe that body or cosmos works like a machine and time is linear. The cosmos is an ever-changing dynamic whole and so is the human body. Time is cyclic. For treatment and cure, body cannot be taken in fragments and an individual should be treated in all physical, mental, social and spiritual contexts.

Role of *karma* in Āyurveda

The role of *karma* is very important in Āyurveda. The results of the past *karma* are called *daiva* and they are responsible in determining the state of health at the time of birth. With the personal effort or present *karma*, called *puruṣakāra*, we can make a given state of health better or worse. There should be a co-ordination between *daiva* and *puruṣakāra* to keep good health. That means we should learn to react according to our own constitution. If we have good health due to our *daiva*, we should not neglect to maintain our health. We should make every effort to maintain that state of well-being which we have due to our previous *karma*. In case we suffer from ill health due to our *daiva*, we should work hard (*puruṣakāra*) to cure ourselves and to restore health.

Āyurveda accords great importance to yogic ways, specifically to the mental equilibrium for good health and longevity. Yogic postures (*yogāsanas*) and breathing practices (*prāṇāyāma*) are recommended for maintaining health, curing ailments, and for spiritual healing. Along with rational therapy, Āyurveda lays a great emphasis on mental and spiritual therapies and these are done with several yogic methods. According to Āyurvedic wisdom, one may be aiming for having physical enjoyment, mental pleasure or for a spiritual goal, but a healthy body is essential in all cases. According to yoga, a healthy, clean and pure body and balanced mind is essential to achieve the aim of yoga. An adept of yoga has to learn to control the senses and mind. This control is achieved through purification practices of the body, breathing exercises, yoga postures and by acquiring the *sattvic* qualities like truth, virtue and equilibrium. It is obvious that an unhealthy body cannot go on the path of yoga. Therefore, in this respect, yoga and Āyurveda merge with each other. Āyurvedic wisdom of maintaining the equilibrium of three main governing forces of the body, enhancing strength and vitality, and healing the ailments with various natural medicines is also essential to learn for an adept of yoga. Involvement with the world is through body and mind and for liberation also, these two are the vehicles. If one is involved with the ailments and troubles of the body, how can one aspire to conquer one's senses?

Āyurveda is a scientific discipline and it aims to achieve perfect physical and mental health, enhance the quality of life and to attain longevity. It does not tell you whether you should use healthy body for worldly pleasures or spiritual goals. It suggests that the first priority of life should be to safeguard your health, the second to have material means to sustain life and the third priority should be to achieve a spiritual goal. Unlike yoga of Patañjali, Āyurveda does not suggest renunciation. Āyurveda provides us with wisdom on sensuous pleasures like sexuality, culinary arts and other pleasures of life to enhance the joy of life.

The other yogas in the context of Patañjali's yoga

Until now, I have basically talked about Patañjali's yoga, which is also referred to as 'the Yoga' because, as mentioned earlier, it is one of the six major schools of thought from ancient India. However, there are also other yogic ways and methods and there are many sub-schools of this discipline. To understand Patañjali and the yogic tradition better, it is essential to comprehend the other yogas and their relationship to Patañjali's yoga. But first of all, let us see the etymology of the word yoga. This word has its root in the Sanskrit word 'yuj', which means to yoke, fasten, join, unite, harness, concentrate the mind on something or to meditate. Some of the other meanings of the word are to make ready, to prepare, to set to work, use and apply. It is said that the word 'yuj' has common roots with the Latin word 'jungere' which means to join, thus giving rise to subsequent words 'jouge' in French, 'joch' in German and 'yoke' in English, which means a frame with which two animals are joined for working together. The word 'yoga' has been used in different scriptures in numerous senses (for details see Monier-Williams, Sanskrit-English Dictionary). Some of the principal meanings are employment, use, application, performance, mixing of different things, arrangement, disposition, regular succession, suitability, endeavour, zeal, diligence, union, contact, connection or mental concentration. The applied philosophical meaning of the word 'yoga' is in the sense of a spiritual discipline, for the purpose of ultimate union of the individual soul with the Universal Soul. The word is also widely used to express the method or technique or employment or application. A derivative of the word yoga is 'viniyoga', which has been used by Patañjali in Sūtra 6, Part III, in the sense of employment or use.

In different sub-schools of yoga, the methods and techniques may differ but the ultimate aim remains the same, that is the submergence of the individual soul into the Universal soul or the absolute.

In the *Bhagavad Gītā,* where Kṛṣṇa is instructing Arjuna on yoga, all the eighteen discourses are named with different yogas using pre-fix before the word yoga. The yoga techniques of the *Bhagavad Gītā* principally centre around *karma,* knowledge and devotion. All these different ways lead to the same goal:

'The one who, with the help of devotion succeeds in knowing My true nature, thus knowing me at last in truth, enters with the prayer into me.'[15]

Kṛṣṇa is the representation of *Brahman* or the Absolute and this *śloka* indicates the fulfilment of the ultimate aim of yoga, the dissolution into the Absolute. Kṛṣṇa shows his cosmic appearance to Arjuna in the eleventh discourse of the *Bhagavad Gītā* and that

15 *Bhagavad Gītā,* XVIII, 55.

makes it clear that he symbolises the Universal Soul.

The word '*Puruṣa*' for *Brahman* was used in Vedas and Upaniṣads as well as in the *Bhagavad Gītā*:

> **'That, the highest *Puruṣa*, may be reached by devotion alone, in whom all beings abide, by whom all this is pervaded.'**[16]

As we see, the yoga of the *Bhagavad Gītā* is principally the yoga through devotion (*Bhakti-yoga*). The personal effort of *karma*-yoga is also to dedicate the fruits of one's actions to the Lord. The Lord may be the Absolute or *Puruṣa* or one of the smaller gods, which provide the stepping stones to reach the higher goal. The *Bhagavad Gītā* recognises that a direct path to attain union with the unembodied *Brahman* is infinitely harder:

> **'The difficulty of those whose minds are set on the unmanifested is greater, for the path of the unmanifested is hard for the embodied to reach.'**[17]

Compared to the *Bhagavad Gītā*, Patañjali's yoga teaches the practices which are largely based upon personal effort than devotion and submission to the Lord. The central emphasis in the *Bhagavad Gītā* is on devotion and on the glory of *Brahman*. Our actions and prayers are attributed to Him to ultimately attain oneness with Him. In Patañjali's yoga, the centre of attention is the individual with intellect, mind and body. Patañjali has described ingeniously the integration of the soul, intellect, mind and body and their relationship with the cosmos. He has shown the techniques of dissociation first from the body, and then from the world in order to find the stillness of mind. Through all this comes the recognition of one's real self, the soul. These are the steps of the ladder to achieve finally the total isolation of the soul (*kaivalya*) from the physical being as well as the phenomenal world. The soul is isolated from its vehicle of action, *Prakrti* and is liberated from it. Unlike in the *Bhagavad Gītā*, Patañjali does not talk about the union of the individual soul with the Universal Soul. This can be understood as follows: *Puruṣa* is bound to action because of its union with *Prakṛti* and when they are isolated by

---

[16] *Bhagavad Gītā*, VIII, 22, In this *śloka*, 'this' (*idam*) refers to *Prakṛti* and 'that' (*tat*) refers to *Puruṣa*.

[17] *Ibid*, XII, 5

the individual through yogic ways, the part of *Puruṣa* in the individual finds union (yoga) with the Eternal *Puruṣa*. In fact, the individual soul is only separated from the Universal Soul as far as it is involved with the phenomenal world and is bound to the cycle of birth and death through *karma*.

Another major difference between the yoga of the *Bhagavad Gītā* and that of Patañjali is that the principal duties (*mahāvrata*) of an adept of yoga for Patañjali are irrespective of his caste, place, period and time. The first of the great duties outlined in Patañjali's eight-fold path is *yama* or restraint. One of the five *yamas* is *ahiṃsā* (not to kill or cause pain to others). Part II, Sūtra 34 of Patañjali's Yogasūtra states:

> **'Questionable acts such as killing etc., whether done, caused to be done or approved of; whether resulting from greed, anger or attachment; whether slight, intermediate or beyond measure, result in endless pain and ignorance and hence should be opposed.'**

This is in contrast to Kṛṣṇa's teachings to Arjuna where the latter must fulfil his duties as a warrior, which is the *dharma* of his caste.[18]

The yoga of Patañjali is considered as the classical yoga and other forms of yoga deal with one or more steps of the eight-fold yogic practices described by him. Patañjali's yoga is also called *Rāja yoga*. The literal meaning of the word is royal or kingly yoga. But in the present context, it is meant entirely in another sense. The word *rāja* is used to describe the state of mind when the adept has a complete control over the activities of his/her mind. The activities of the mind are controlled by the mind itself. Thus, the mind in this case is the king or the governing agent to control its own activities and these latter are not governed by the senses, which are constantly attracted to the phenomenal world. The mind is the master and its authority is used to subjugate the senses.

Haṭha yoga or the yoga of hardness (yoga for making oneself tough) deals with making body stronger with purification practices, *yogāsanas* and *prāṇāyāma* (breathing practices). All these practices are a part of Patañjali's eight-fold yoga. In fact, in the two major texts of *Haṭha yoga* (*Haṭha Yoga Pradīpikā* and *Gheraṇḍa Saṃhitā*), it is mentioned in the opening verse that *Haṭha yoga*

---

[18] *Bhagavad Gītā*, II, 31-33

is taught as a preparation for *Rāja yoga* and that it is the first step of the ladder leading to *Rāja yoga.*

The word 'yoga' seems to have enigmatic qualities as in our times also, it is very widely used in many senses. I have seen and heard expressions like 'Chinese yoga', 'Christian yoga' and so on. Sometimes, this word is used to describe a difficult physical posture and at other times, it is used for a sort of mental concentration or inner discipline also from other cultures. In fact, all religions teach methods to achieve self-discipline and mental stillness.

Tāntric tradition

It is important to consider the other parallel currents of thoughts, which had a tremendous influence later on the previous disciplines and gave rise to hybridisation. The *Tāntric* principles and practices have had a tremendous influence on the philosophical and religious tradition of India. This tradition was developed through ages and was adopted by Hindus, Buddhists and Jainas. It is thought that the *Tāntric* principles were well established in India by the second century BC. :

> **'...although the first *Tantras* and the first Yoga Upanishads, for instance, date from eight century after Christ, we may and should assume as a certainty that their contents were formulated at least ten centuries earlier, then continuously elaborated upon and renewed before being finally fixed in the texts we possess.'**[19]

Some thinkers believe that the earlier codified *Tāntric* texts date back from the beginning of the Christian era if not earlier.

> **'...several *Tantric* texts have been found written in Sanskrit Gupta characters which establish their date as AD 400-600; in addition, there exist manuscripts of Saiva Agamas from South India from the sixth century.'**[20]

In the *Tāntric* tradition, the Lord and his creative power *Śakti* represent *Puruṣa* and *Prakṛti*. They are considered as a God and

[19] Jean Varenne, 1976, *Yoga and the Hindu Tradition,* The University of Chicago Press, Chicago, p. 182.

[20] Ajit Mookerji and Madhu Khanna, 1977, *The Tantric Way,* New York Graphic Society, Boston, p. 10.

a Goddess. In various schools of this tradition, the God is Viṣṇu or Śiva and his consort Lakṣmī or Pārvatī. Thus, the relationship between *Puruṣa* and *Prakṛti* has evolved to be a relationship of male and female. One of the meanings of the word *'Puruṣa'* is male or man and the word *'Prakṛti'* means nature and it is feminine in gender. The human body is the microcosmos of the macrocosmos and the existence is signified by the cohabitation of male and female principles. These principles in *Tāntric* tradition are *ātman* and *kuṇḍalinī. Ātman* (soul) is a part of the Lord and *kuṇḍalinī* is the *Śakti* representing the Goddess. The word *kuṇḍalinī* literally means coiled over itself. *Kuṇḍalinī* is represented by various signs and symbols such as fire or a serpent and it lies in dormant form in the human body. The aim of tantra yoga is to awake this dormant power. The ultimate aim is achieved by dissolution (*laya*) of the risen power of *kuṇḍalinī* into *ātman.*

Within the human body, there lies a subtle body called *sūkśmaśarīra.* The subtle body is represented by a network of *nāḍīs* or channels and it is compared to the universe itself. Various elements of the cosmos are represented in different parts of the body. The *prāṇa* or the cosmic vitality is guided into different parts of the subtle body through the *nāḍīs* . The three principal *nāḍīs* are *iḍā, piṅgalā* and *suṣumnā. Suṣumnā nāḍī* is straight and is in the middle of the back whereas *iḍā* and *piṅgalā* cross *suṣumnā* at six different places. The intersections of the three *nāḍīs* at six places represent six of the seven major *cakras.* One of the meanings of the word *cakra* is wheel but here it indicates the confluent point of vital energy, which is circulated around. Different *cakras* are the steps of the ladder for the rise of the *kuṇḍalinī* energy. The seventh *cakra* is located on the top of the head and indicates the termination of the journey of *kuṇḍalinī* and its meeting with the *ātman.* At this state, the adept becomes one with *Brahman* and is liberated from the cycle of birth and death, *saṃsāra.* In Figure 6, the names of the *cakras,* their location, sound and activity are summarized.

Advaita and yoga

The diverse doctrines with variation in their approach have the same goal, dissolution of the self into the Absolute for attaining freedom from the cycle of birth and death. The *advaita* (non-dualism) *Vedānta* doctrine of *Śaṃkara* (788-820 AD) emphasises the

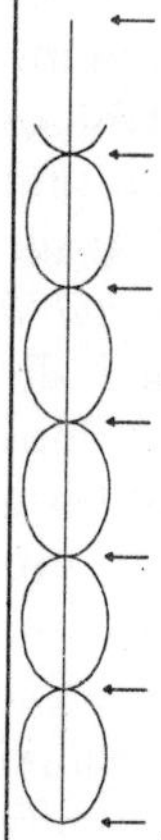

Location In the Body	Name	Symbolic Sound: Mantra	Element	Vital Activity
Top of the head	*Sahasrāra*	Beyond all sounds; denotes the Universal Soul	Universal Soul	Beyond all activities
Between eyebrows	*Ājñā*	*OṂ*	Mind	Mental function
Throat	*Viśuddha*	*Haṃ*	Ether	Hearing
Plexus	*Anāhata*	*Yaṃ*	Air	Touch
Navel	*Maṇipūra*	*Raṃ*	Fire	Sight
Genitals	*Svādhiṣṭhāna*	*Vaṃ*	Water	Taste
Anus	*Mūlādhāra*	*Laṃ*	Earth	Smell

Figure 6. A diagrammatic representation of the three principal channels of the subtle body and location of the concentric energy points or *cakras*. The name, sound (mantra), their corresponding elements and vital activity of each *cakra* are also given.

non-dualism of *Puruṣa* and *Prakṛti* and postulates a single ultimate reality, the *Brahman.* The phenomenal world is considered to be a delusion, *māyā,* which accounts for a variety of things in the manifest world when in reality all is one. *Brahman* pervades the universe but its presence is inferred only from its effect. If we look at the *Sāṃkhya* table (Table 2), we do realise that only with the union of *Puruṣa* and *Prakṛti* does the individuating principle (*ahaṃkāra*) arise and the whole cosmos is the product of that.

According to *Vedānta, māyā* operates in the mind of the individual and causes ignorance or *avidyā.* That means that the individual takes the phenomenal world for real. This is not different from Patañjali's view, according to which the root cause of our afflictions is *avidyā.* It is due to *avidyā* that we consider the phenomenal world as eternal, pure and joyful (*Yogasūtra,* Part II, Sūtra 5). The principal difference between *Sāṃkhya* and *Vedānta* is that the former emphasises upon the individual soul whereas in *Vedānta* of *Śaṃkara*, oneness of all souls is considered. It is said that the individual souls are like reflection of moon in different buckets of water. The reflection does not change the reality of the moon, which is one. I will not go further in details on this theme, as our aim here is to apply the ancient wisdom of yoga and Āyurveda in our daily lives and not to get into the speculative controversies amongst various schools of thought.

Cosmos, phenomenal world and the gods

Some scholars wrongly interpret that the phenomenal world is denied in the Hindu tradition. It should be clearer to the reader that for the Hindus, the manifest world is only one part of the multidimensional and multi-layered reality. There are other dimensions of reality which are not manifested. The physical self is not denied but it is emphasised that it is not only the body, which is the self of an individual. The body, mind and intellect are described in the following hierarchical order. The senses are great but greater than the senses is the mind. Greater than the mind is intellect or power to discriminate, the *buddhi*, and even greater is the soul that is the cause of being and is a part of the eternal reality. It is stressed in all schools and sub-schools of thought that the real experiencer is the soul along with the body, senses, mind and intellect. In *Kaṭha Upaniṣad*, this relationship is described as follows:

> **'Body is like a chariot, of which soul is the owner,**
> **the intellect is the driver,**
> **the mind plays the part of reins,**
> **senses are the horses,**
> **and the world is their arena.'**[21]

Thus, we see that for proceeding towards any aim, the chariot (body) should be in the best of conditions. The command is given by the intellect and the control is exercised by the mind. Horses are the driving force for the chariot and so are the senses for existence in this world. The energy that holds together all these dimensions of being is the soul, the owner of the chariot. This makes clear that the sensuous part of the existence is very

---

21 *Kaṭha Upaniṣad*, III, 3-4.

important in the Hindu worldview as no chariot can run without horses. However, the wild horses without any control will also bring the chariot to ruin. The control of the mind over the senses through intellect is the important message.

Because of the cosmic oneness and interrelationship of all that exists, the Hindus respect and venerate the multiple dimensions of the cosmic reality. This explains why Hindus worship the great rivers, sun, moon, planets, stars, and why there are gods of wind, love and lust. It also gives answer to why the earth is worshipped before and after the crop and before beginning the construction of a house and other such ceremonies. Human beings are a part of the larger cosmic energy and to emphasise the human connection with the other cosmic energies, various natural phenomena are personified in different gods. The personification makes them similar to human beings but their godly status depicts their greater strength than we have. The worship and veneration of all these gods with offerings, mantras, meditation and so on is to show human gratitude and respect to them as life giving forces and to emphasise the idea of cosmic unity and interdependence.

Gods in their personifications have philosophical symbolism. The trident of Śiva is symbolic of the three qualities of *Prakṛti* (*sattva, rajas, tamas*). The snake around his neck represents time and destruction related to time. Śiva is also called the god of time, *kāleśvara.* The tiger skin he sits on represents desire (Figure 7).

Goddess Kālī is a symbol of power or *śakti* and also symbolises *kāla* or time. In fact, it represents the power of time that constantly changes everything. The garland of human heads around her neck symbolises wisdom, her red tongue signifies *rajas,* the quality which gives impetus to all activities. The sword and the severed head in her hand signify *karma* (Figure 8).

Śivaliṅga in *yoni* pedestal symbolises the union of the male and female organs in their cosmic totality (Figure 9).

Kṛṣṇa with his consort Rādhā and the magic of his flute represent the *Puruṣa, Prakṛti* and the phenomenal world (Figure 10).

I hope that this brief account of the vast Hindu tradition will help you to understand yoga and Āyurveda in their proper perspective and also in the living tradition of the Hindus. For the application of both, yoga and Āyurveda in your daily lives, it is important to first understand the concept of body in the Hindu tradition and the holistic worldview of the ancient sages of this

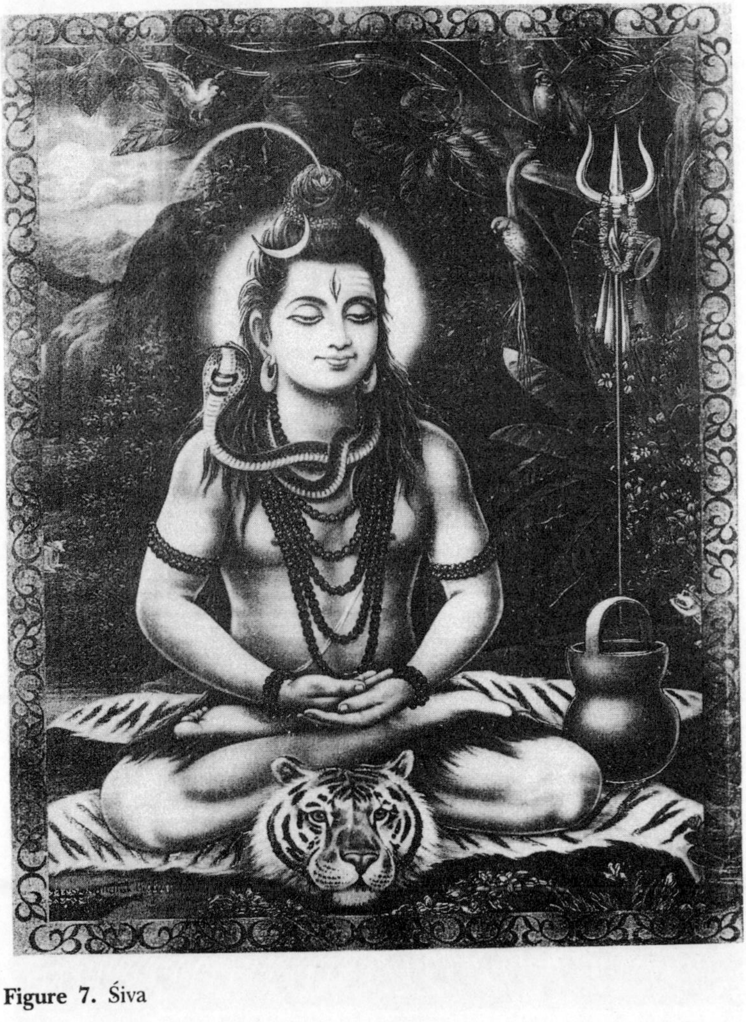

Figure 7. Śiva

continent. The modern human beings are conditioned to a fragmented approach to life and therefore it is essential for the understanding of these ancient Indian doctrines to be able to see the cosmos as a united whole.

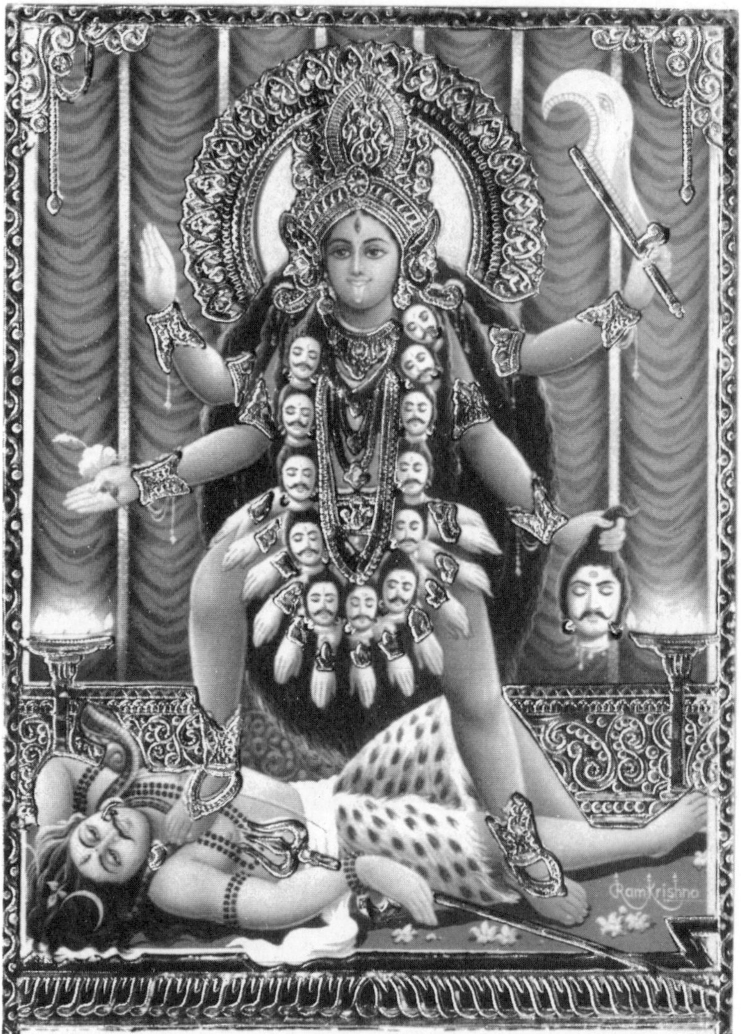

Figure 8. Kālī

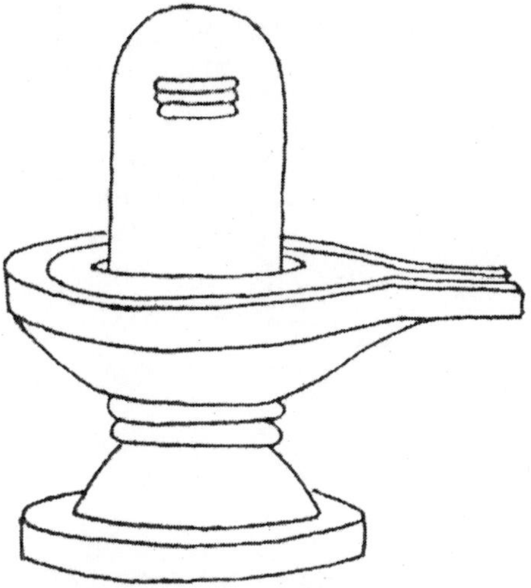

Figure 9. *Śivaliṅga* in *yoni*

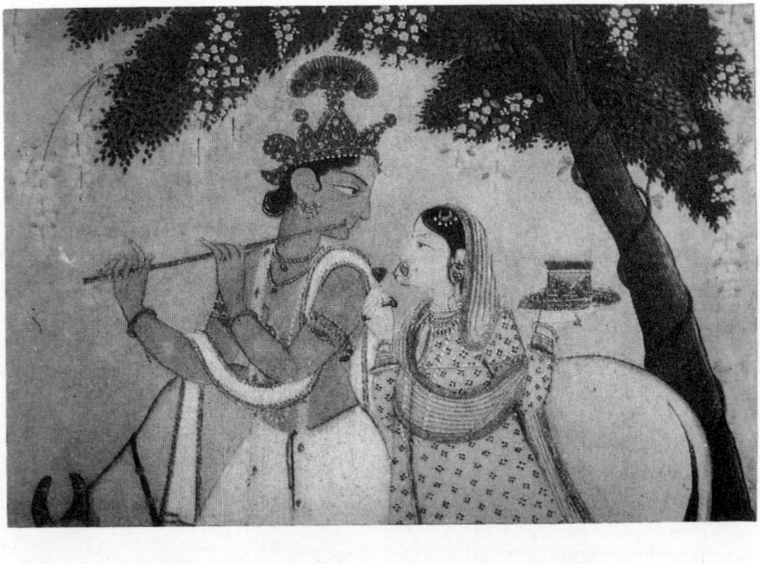

Figure 10. Kṛṣṇa with his flute and his consort Rādhā

SECTION II

Yogasūtra of Patañjali and Their Timeless Wisdom

In the previous Section, you have already had a brief introduction to the *Yogasūtra* of Patañjali. In this Section, we will go into the details of the text of the *Yogasūtra* so that you can comprehend how this timeless wisdom is important for our daily lives. The *Yogasūtra* are however for a specific aim, that is liberation from the cycle of birth and death and to attain eternity by being one with the ultimate reality of the universe. We will see that to reach the ultimate goal, one has to master many techniques to acquire a complete physical and mental well-being and a high energy level. These various techniques are invaluable for us in the context of Āyurvedic yoga, a term which I have coined after having studied Patañjali and the major Āyurvedic texts, particularly *Caraka Saṃhitā*.

The Essence of the *Yogasūtra*

Before going into the details of the Sūtras, let us have an overview of the central theme of the *Yogasūtra*. If I have to convey the central theme of Patañjali's text in very simple words, I would put it as follows:

We human beings are extremely involved with our pains and pleasures. Our physical existence or life span is only for a limited period but somehow, we love the idea of its being permanent. This idea enhances our pain further as in this world all is temporary and transitory. We think that our reality is our physical self and we consider that as our identity. There is something more to our existence than our physical self; that is an invisible energy in us, which makes the physical body alive. This energy is indestructible and immortal and it is our real self. This real self or soul is in fact our continuity in the cosmos. When one physical body expires, this energy becomes the cause of life in another body and thus our real self continues to exist. The inability to distinguish the immortal real self from the ephemeral physical self is unwise and leads to suffering. We learn, we earn, we accumulate different means of comfort and pleasure for us. We indulge in various sensuous pleasures and

gradually, we have to give up all these due to old age and finally death. However, an individual's continuity is soul, which leaves the body at the time of death and acquires a new body in due course of time. The quality of the next life (health, wealth, education, and type of family etc.) depends upon the results of the previous *karma*. The sum total of the remains of previous *karma* in the form of *saṃskāra* also determines our personality. The cycle of life and death goes on forever.

The path of liberation from the cycle of birth and death and to gain immortality is in following steps:

1. **To recognise one's real self, soul and get completely uninvolved from the physical and the ephemeral.**
2. **Bring the mind to complete stillness by stopping the thought process and this way the mind gets uninvolved with world. A thought-free mind acquires the nature of the soul and is no more the doer of the *karma*.**
3. **By continuous and repeated practice of the above (no. 2), the adept is able to dissolve the previous *karma* and can reach a state of non-performance of further *karma*.**
4. **A continuity of the above state (no. 3) leads to a complete separation of the cause of being, the soul from its vehicle, the body.**
5. **When this separation occurs, the soul gets completely free from its vehicle, the body, and becomes one with the Universal Soul. It gets out of the cycle of birth and death. A yogī does not die a natural death like the other human beings. He or she 'leaves the body' at a chosen time. The soul of the yogī is a lready integrated into *Puruṣa* or the Universal Soul.**

This was the single-page essence of the *Yogasūtra*. In the following pages, we will go in more details of the techniques that Patañjali has described extremely logically. Patañjali is a great scientist of all times and his 195 Sūtras must have been the result of tremendous amount of research in profoundness of human mind, cosmic reality and the existence itself. When I use the word 'scientist' for Patañjali, I do not mean, as it is understood in the sense of modern science, which is limited to the material or sensuous reality of the cosmos.

Patañjali's Exposition of Yoga

The book that has 195 Sūtras or aphorisms is divided into four Parts. The Part I is on the Exposition of Meditation and contains 51 Sūtras. The Part II is on the Exposition of Practice and the Part III is on the Exposition of Accomplishments and each has 55 Sūtras. The Part IV is on the Exposition of the Absolute Isolation and has 34 Sūtras.

The Part I is on the following theme:

1. Working of the human mind and its qualities.
2. The difference between the meditative and non-meditative states of mind.
3. The hindrance in the way of attaining meditation and the methods to remove them.
4. Different ways of attaining steadiness of the mind and finally different stages of the meditative mind before it reaches the final state of the absolute isolation.

Let us see all these in more detail.

EXPOSITION OF THE MEDITATION (PART I)

There is always a chain of thoughts in our mind. One thought leads to another and it is a never-ending process. Even during our sleep, when our senses are inert, the mind continues with its thinking process at another level. For example, we have dreams during sleep. Even if we do not have dreams or are not able to recall them upon waking up, we are nevertheless aware of the quality of sleep we have had.

Citta is the thinking principle of the mind and its *vṛtti* or the intrinsic quality is to undergo constant modifications. To hinder this intrinsic quality of the thinking principle of the mind and bring it to attain a thought-free state is yoga. Patañjali gives this definition of yoga in the second Sūtra of Part I (*Yogaścittavṛtti-nirodhaḥ*). I will give a detailed explanation of this definition of yoga.

Through our five senses, we are constantly perceiving the world of sound, touch, form, taste and smell. The mind processes that new knowledge, accumulates it and the thoughts are the combination of the past and present sensuous experiences as well as the fantasies and fears about the future. Let me take a simple example to illustrate that. You happen to listen to a song that used to be very popular during your childhood. That reminds you of one of your classmates who used to sing that particular song. Then you begin to think about this person—that she was a brilliant student but she did not continue her studies and got married after school. And this reminds you of one of your teachers who used to appreciate this friend of yours and was very sorry for her discontinuing the studies. Then you remember an incident of last year when you happened to meet this particular teacher on a train station fifteen years after having left the school. You were returning from your vacations and when you saw this familiar face, you stopped for a while and then recollected who he was. Meanwhile, he had turned all grey and you took time to recognise him. This thought takes you to last year's vacation and like this the thought process goes on. We are mostly unaware of the link of one thought to the other and go on throughout life with the chain of thoughts. For Descartes, this process was existence itself but for Patañjali, by hindering this process, we discover the profoundness of human capabilities.

What happens when we hinder the thinking process with a conscious effort? To understand this, we need to comprehend the relationship of senses, mind, intellect and soul.

Through the five senses, the phenomenal world is constantly perceived by the mind. Thus, the mind undergoes continuous modifications. The living element in the body or the cause of all these phenomena of the senses and the mind is soul. The soul does not undergo any modification. It is not involved with the activities of the mind and it is like a reflecting glass. It reflects the state of mind in it. Just as a moving object will give a turbulent reflection and a still object will reflect a still image, similar is the situation of mind and soul. The mind is constantly undergoing modifications and that is its basic nature as it operates through senses, which perceive and absorb constantly the ever-changing dynamic, attractive and beautiful phenomenal world. Human mind has also a power of discrimination or *buddhi*. The *buddhi* has the ability to discern and control the activities of the mind and thus, human beings can discriminate about their sensuous involvement with the world. Despite the fact that the mind's intrinsic quality is to constantly modify, it is also capable of controlling itself. Through this power of mind, the senses can be liberated from the world and the mind can be brought to stillness by intercepting the chain of thoughts. When the mind is thought-free and still, it acquires the nature of the soul, which is pure energy, is still, is not involved with the activities of the world and is a part of the cosmic energy—the *Puruṣa.* The oneness of the individual soul with the cosmic energy is the state of yoga. In other words, a meditative mind is thought-free and still and acquires the nature of the soul. A non-meditative mind, which is undergoing modifications, is involved in the world through the senses and its activities are reflected by the soul. This idea of meditative and non-meditative states of mind is illustrated in Figure 11.

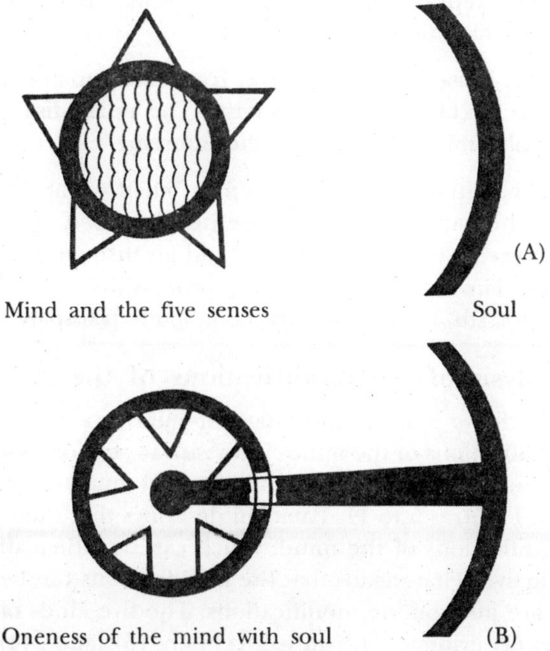

Figure 11. (A) The mind is constantly getting new knowledge through five senses and is undergoing modifications. The soul is simply an onlooker and is aloof.

(B) The senses are closed to the world and the mind has stopped the modifications and is still. The mind without modifications acquires the nature of the soul and this is the state of the meditative mind.

Before we proceed further, it is important to clarify that non-involvement of the senses does not mean simply shutting them. Some people take vows of not speaking or they use some sort of penance to withdraw their senses, but with the methods described by Patañjali, the non-involvement is with the control of mind and is achieved by repeated practice. Persons who try to withdraw their senses simply by not speaking or closing their eyes and repeating a mantra but their mind is wandering, are not able to achieve the stillness of mind. Kṛṣṇa has emphasised the same in the *Bhagavad Gītā*:

> **"Like a tortoise that withdraws its limbs from all directions, the adept of yoga withdraws the senses from the sense objects and his mind attains stability.**
>
> **The sense objects turn away from that who does not enjoy them but the taste for them persists. This relish disappears when the stable-minded visualises the Supreme."**[1]

We may function with the senses but if we are uninvolved with the phenomenal world, we are not disturbed by the happenings. The events of the world come and go through the vehicle of our body. The senses and the mind process the happenings but these do not stir us as if we are completely transparent.

Analysis of the modifications of the mind

To achieve a meditative state of mind, we need to hinder the modifications of the mind. If we wish to stop or hinder something, we must understand its nature and qualities beforehand. In Part I, Sūtras 5 to 11, Patañjali describes that there are five major modifications of the mind, which can be either afflictive or non-afflictive. That means that the modifications can be either painful or are just routine modifications. The five kinds of modifications are: (1) evidence, (2) misconception, (3) fancy, (4) sleep and (5) memory.

1. **Evidence:** We perceive something through our senses. The object perceived is imprinted on our mind with its form, colour, smell etc. The second step is that the mind cognises that image of the object and infers its identity (whether it

---

[1] *Bhagavadgītā*, II, 58-59.

is a river, a mountain, a cow, a tree or a table and so on). The inference depends upon testimony. I call a stone a stone or a tree a tree because others before me have done it. It is important to understand that these three steps of modification of the mind are distinct from each other. I perceive a table and infer it according to the previous knowledge that it is a table. My perception is different from the reality of the table. They are two distinct things. I call this thing with four legs and a flat top a table because others before me have decided to do so. I distinguish a table from a bed although they are similar in their fundamental form but different in shape and size. That means that I have certain beliefs as what a table should be and what a bed should be.

All this may sound like an unnecessary discussion to some of you, but it is important at this stage to comprehend these differences in order to achieve the stillness of the mind. When these three stages of evidence become one for a person, the mind attains stillness. For example if I fix my mind on the reality of the table, that is, the mass, shape and form of the table forgetting about its name and image in my mind, the first step is achieved to hinder the modifications of the mind. Try this exercise with different objects around you and you will have this experience. For example, go to a quiet garden, stay at a fair distance from a tree and just concentrate on the form of the tree forgetting all about its name and other knowledge about it. That means, you are only visually absorbing the form of the tree and are not letting your mind wander about inferring and testifying this sensuous experience of visualising a tree. This is a very simple method to attain a thought-free mind at least for a short interval.

2. **Misconception:** It is an incorrect notion that does not reveal the real nature of the object concerned. This modification of the mind may occur at various levels. One may mistake a strong night-light for moon, plastic plants for the real ones, mirage of the desert for water and so on. At another level, one may interpret the noise of leaves for a tiger while walking in the forest. Some fainted person may be mistaken for dead and an already dead person may be considered

as still alive. To believe the false as truth and what is real and true as false is another example of mistaken notion or misconception.

3. **Fancy:** This is the knowledge conveyed by words and is devoid of an object. Thoughts like imagination about the future, heaven, hell, projecting oneself to be rich, fearing oneself to be poor and so on are in this category. The abstract concepts like '*Puruṣa* and *Prakṛti* together are the cause of phenomenal world', 'our future is decided from our past and present *karma*', 'the universe is an ever-changing and dynamic whole' and so on, are the modifications of the mind which come in the category of fancy.
4. **Sleep:** It is that modification, which occurs in the absence of new knowledge as the senses are temporarily closed to the external world during sleep. All the sense organs and organs of action are in an inert stage during sleep. However, the modifications of the mind go on during sleep. There are dreams during sleep, which can be recalled after waking up. Even if one may think that the sleep was without dreams, one is still aware of the kind of sleep one had like sound sleep, restless sleep etc. The mental processes do not stop during sleep despite the fact that the sensory perception is considerably reduced. I have used the word 'reduced', as it is not totally closed because during sleep, if there is a loud noise or a strong smell or too much light or someone touches us, we wake up.
5. **Memory:** It is the retention of notion we have already had. Due to memory, our thought process is constantly occupied. It is my theory that we never forget anything. Everything is stored in our minds but certain memories are suppressed or stacked in the profounder layers. For example, when we see a person, who was with us in the kindergarten or primary school thirty years ago, our mind starts to search and tries to place that known face. We generally end up recognising and remembering the person concerned. Besides this kind of dormant memory, we have active thoughts from the recent past. Thus, our mind is often occupied with events, which are based on memory and this modification of mind along with the present perception makes the regular chain of thoughts in the mind.

Pain and pleasure from the five modifications

The five kinds of modifications of the mind are either afflictive or non-afflictive. They may bring us pain or may not bring us pain. In fact, whether they bring us pain or pleasure in the normal sense of the world, they will come under the category of afflictive. The material and sensuous pleasures do not remain constant in this ever-changing dynamic world. The departure of pleasure is also pain. In the present context, non-afflictive will be those modifications of the mind, which lead one to wisdom of recognising one's real self, soul as distinct from the destructible and perishable physical self. I will deal with this theme in more detail a little later as Patañjali has described the details of affliction in Part II of the *Yogasūtra.*

Why and how to stop the modifications of the mind?

It has been briefly said earlier about the aim of Patañjali's yoga. The purpose of an ordinary, worldly human being may be different from the adept of yoga who is working to achieve liberation and eternity. However, in the present context of Āyurvedic yoga, we are aiming to achieve mental and physical strength and to develop healing capabilities with the initiation into the discipline of yoga. I will deal with the practical aspects of this in the last section of the book.

Whatever the purpose, to stop the modifications of the mind is a very tough task. In *Bhagavad Gītā,* Kṛṣṇa preached Arjuna about the importance of yoga and Arjuna asked the following to Kṛṣṇa:

> **'The yoga which you have described with such facility, I do not see it practical because of the ever-changing nature of the mind. The mind is very unsteady, turbulent, tenacious and powerful and therefore I consider that restraining it is as unfeasible as controlling the wind.'[2]**

There are two key things in Kṛṣṇa's reply to Arjuna for controlling the mind—repeated practice and detachment[3]. In Sūtra 12 of Part I, Patañjali has said the same: 'Hindering the modifications

---

[2] *Bhagavadgītā,* VI, 33-34.
[3] *Ibid,* VI, 35.

of the mind is accomplished by repeated practice and dispassion.' An endeavour is to be made again and again to reduce the mind to a condition of freedom from modifications. Each time a thought penetrates the mind, one has to remind oneself to get rid of it. One thought gives rise to another and a chain is formed. Therefore, one should be very strict with oneself. Various techniques to achieve a thought-free mind are told in Part II of the *Yogasūtra.*

'Dispassion is to attain the consciousness of not thirsting after objects either seen or heard of' (Part I, Sūtra 15). Worldly things like a house, land, wealth or other human beings are the 'object seen'. 'Objects heard of' are those about which knowledge is obtained through scriptures or other sources. Dispassion gives rise to the knowledge of the cause of being—the *Puruṣa.*
Patañjali has suggested the path of yoga in the following sequence:

1. **Devotion:** One should be dedicated to the cause of yoga, that is, to attain freedom from the cycle of life and death. With this aim, one automatically feels detached from the perishable worldly objects and passions.
2. **Energy:** Devotion, as described above, gives rise to energy to pursue the cause with enthusiasm and perseverance.
3. **Memory:** This step helps to remind oneself of the aim and to remain alert to attain a thought-free mind. For example, if we sit still and do *prāṇāyāma* or the breathing practices and then repeat a mantra (*japa*) to attain a thought-free mind, the thoughts may creep in nevertheless. One has to stand on guard not to let the thoughts come to mind and should remember to dissolve oneself in the mantra.
4. **Meditation:** By repeating persistently step 3, one achieves a meditative state of mind. The thought-free mind is in the state of stillness and acquires the nature of the soul.
5. **Discernment:** Step 4 leads to self-realisation, that is, the recognition of one's real self, soul as distinct from the physical, ephemeral body.

There are variations from one individual to the other in attaining the meditative state of mind. Even amongst those, who are rapid, there are further variations (Part I, Sūtra 21-22). We notice tremendous individual variation in intelligence, ability to assimilate, ability to concentrate, creativity and so on and this evidently is also applicable for achieving a thought-free mind.

Sūtras 23 to 29 of Part I are devoted to an alternative way of attaining meditation. A profound devotion to *Īśvara* helps attain meditation. This Sūtra, taken out of context, has led Patañjali's critics to say that he is theistic as one of the meanings of the word '*Īśvara*' is also god. I have two counter arguments to this criticism. Firstly, the word *Īśvara* does not only mean god. In common language, this word does denote the embodied God, but in the ancient literature, it also signifies *Brahman* or the Universal Soul, which is the *Puruṣa* of *Sāṃkhya* and yoga. In *Īśa Upaniṣad*, it is described as follows:

'It encircles all things,
radiant and bodiless,
unharmed and untouched by evil,
all seeing, all wise,
all present, self-existent'.[4]

Let me give you the text of the seven Sūtras (23-29) below and you will realise that Patañjali does not mean the embodied God by *Īśvara* as he clarifies himself about this word and its significance in the present context.

'A profound devotion to *Īśvara* also helps attain meditation. *Īśvara* is defined as that which is untouched by afflictions, actions and their fruits and the consequent desires produced by them. It is the guru of even the earlier created beings, as it is not bound by time. Its appellation is *praṇava* or the word OṂ. Its repetition and reflection on its significance destroy all obstacles and bring consciousness of the omnipresent.'

The writer himself states so clearly what he meant by *Īśvara* and specifically when he says that 'it is not bound by time', which leaves no doubt that he refers to *Puruṣa.* Furthermore, Patañjali gives the symbolic significance of *Īśvara* as the syllable OṂ. Viewing all this, to designate *Yogasūtra* as theistic is merely an irresponsible intellectual error. It is possible to make this error if one reads only this Sūtra out of the 195 Sūtras written by the author, because the author repeatedly says about the ultimate aim of yoga which is to isolate one's real self, soul from the physical, ephemeral self. The theme of the *Yogasūtra* is that when the soul is completely

---

[4] *Īśa Upaniṣad,* 8.

isolated, it becomes automatically the part of the *Puruṣa* or the Universal Soul or the Absolute. This will be clearer to you in the rest of this Section as Patañjali has put his basic idea in many different ways throughout his text.

Let us see the significance of OṂ, which has the following figurative form described in Figure 12.

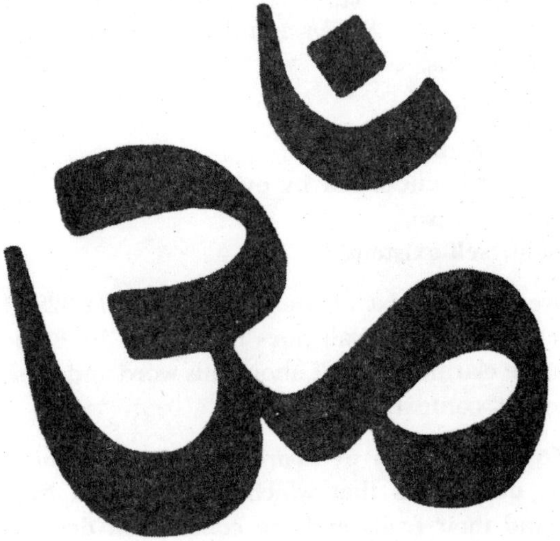

Figure 12. The figurative form of the syllable OṂ, representing the cosmic reality. It has two parts. The bigger lower part signifies the variety and diversity in the phenomenal world. While chanting, it is denoted by a long 'AU...'. The upper part is a crescent with a dot in it and it signifies that despite diversity, all is dissolved into one universe reality, which is the cause of being. This part is chanted by nasal ṃ.

The syllable OṂ is the symbol of the Universal Soul. The first part of the sound is AU..... and it signifies the diversity of the universe. In the figurative form, the whole form except the half moon represents this diversity. There are many colours, shapes, forms, sounds, vegetation, human beings and other animals. There is attractive and fascinating nature with all its diversity. There are mountains, rivers, lakes, oceans, the sun, the moon, stars, day, night and so on. There is happiness, pain, fascination, disgust, wars, misery, hunger and much more. All this diversity dissolves into oneness, that is, the cause of being. It is That which breathes life into the fascinating phenomenal world of diversity. That is the *Puruṣa* and is represented by the half moon and the point in the figurative form of OṂ. In sound, it is the long, nasal ṃ... The repeated pronunciation of the OṂ with the understanding of its significance is called *praṇava.* OṂ is the smallest mantra as it symbolises the cosmos itself. It is very powerful as its pronunciation in an appropriate way or singing also involves the control over respiration (*prāṇāyāma*). The details of the respiration techniques are given in the later part of this Section.

From Sūtra 30 to 39 Patañjali describes the obstacles in the way of yoga and means to combat them. I have made a table of thirteen obstacles and eight means to combat them as has been described by Patañjali in these ten Sūtras (See Table 4). It is interesting to note that for combating the distraction of the mind, Patañjali has given us the choice as there is 'or' after each suggestion. Some of these need more explanation as they are very practical techniques to obtain a thought-free mind and we would be using these techniques in the practice of Āyurvedic yoga.

'Dwelling on a single truth' may mean OṂ representing the ultimate reality or it could be sun, moon, some energy point or *cakra* inside the body or a specific holy place in nature like Mount Kailash.

The second means to combat distraction is to have an attitude of friendship and compassion for all and be satisfied and remain indifferent to happiness, sorrow, virtue or non-virtue. This attitude helps combat distraction by purifying the mind.

Controlled expelling and restraining of the vital energy or breath is called *prāṇāyāma.* It is a highly efficient technique to break the chain of thoughts and bring the mind to stillness. We will discuss the practice of these techniques in the last Part of this book.

Production of sensuous cognition means to concentrate on an intense sensuous experience and this takes out all the other thoughts from mind. By repeating and prolonging this experience, one can prolong the steady state of mind. An intensive experience can be as commonplace as an intensive smell of a flower, beautiful colours of fire, an exclusive sunset or any other sensuous experience that involves us strongly. Music is another example in this category and is most commonly used to attain a thought-free mind in the living tradition of the Hindus. Yoga reveals to us the knowledge about inner self-discipline and in the living tradition, its principles and methods are not only used for the purpose of attaining eternal freedom but also for the peace and strength of the mind. The most common form is *kīrtana,* which is done by repeatedly singing some lines or verses of poetry. It is done in a group. The repetition, tone and music give rise to the intensive sensuous cognition of the sense of hearing. In addition to that, there is devotion involved in this singing. The classical vocal music of India, devotional or otherwise, has a very meditative quality because of harmony and repetition.

A sorrow-free enlightened mind means a state of mind in which *sattva, rajas* and *tamas* are in perfect equilibrium. That means that any event or happening in the world do not disturb one.

A steady state of mind can also be achieved by reflecting upon someone devoid of passion like a great yogī. There are also persons who lead normal worldly life and do their duties for their family and society but they are detached from the world. These are called *karmayogīs* and they can also be inspiring for this purpose.

An effort to relive the state of sleep or dream during wakeful state helps one to achieve the stillness of mind. During sleep, the senses are closed to the external world and thus one achieves the first step and concentrating upon the state of sleep or dream ultimately leads to a thought-free mind.

In the last and eighth means to combat distraction, Patañjali says that one can ponder upon anything one approves of. When we like something, we feel very involved with it and we can easily plunge ourselves in this object. It could be a poem, a piece of music or a statue of a god we are devoted to or anything else.

When the modifications of the mind are weakened with repeated practice, the mind becomes lucid and is capable of seeing distinctly the perceiver (soul), perception (sense organs) and the perceivable (cosmos made of five elements). The reality of these three does not muddle together in a lucid mind.

In the last ten Sūtras of Part I, Patañjali tells us about the five stages of meditation.

The first stage is of argumentative meditative mind. It is achieved by concentrating on an object, for example, sun, with

Table 4. Obstacles in the way of meditation and means to combat them

Obstacles in the way of obtaining steadiness of the mind	**Means to combat these obstacles or distractions of the mind**
1. **Sickness:** Mental or physical imbalance 2. **Languor:** A lack of initiative and enthusiasm about yoga 3. **Doubt:** Hesitation about the practicability of yoga 4. **Carelessness:** A lack of attentiveness to obtain a state of abstraction 5. **Laziness:** Heaviness of mind and body and lack of initiative 6. **Attachment:** A desire for worldly pleasures 7. **Mistaken notions:** Mis-taking some *siddhis* with the ultimate aim of the yoga 8. **Lack of concentration:** Inability to achieve a steady state of mind 9. **Instability:** Repeated discontinuity of the state of concentration or body posture (*āsana*) 10. **Grief:** Thoughts troubling the mind 11. **Distress:** Mental pain due to lack of fulfilment of the desires 12. **Trembling:** Shaking of whole body which prevents steadiness of mind 13. **Sighing:** It is an excessive intake of the air in the body	1. Dwelling upon a single truth: concentrating the mind on the Absolute or 2. Friendship, compassion, tenderness and indifference equally towards happy and unhappy, kind and unkind human beings or 3. Practice of *prāṇāyāma* or 4. Production of sensuous cognition or 5. Obtaining a sorrow-free enlightened mind or 6. Reflection on someone devoid of passion or 7. Dwelling upon dream and sleep knowledge or 8. Pondering upon anything one approves of

the related knowledge of its shape, size, distance etc. The object is the seed of meditation and the concentration gives rise to a meditative stage, which mixes up word, meaning and its knowledge and is bound by these three.

The second and the higher stage of meditation is non-argumentative and the mind is free of the word as the seed of meditation and the conventional sense attached to it. In the present example, only the form of the sun will remain in mind.

The next stage of meditation is called deliberative and the concentration is on the subtle form of the object. In the present example, the subtle form of the sun is light.

Then comes the stage of non-deliberative meditative mind and concentration goes beyond the subtle form of the object. It is beyond space and time and is free from memory, word, meaning, knowledge etc. During all these four stages of meditation, there was an object of concentration (sun in the present example) and therefore they are called the meditation with a seed.

The fifth and the final stage of meditation is without seed and it is when all the previous and present *saṃskāra* are destroyed, the soul abides in its own nature, and is completely isolated from the physical, material, ephemeral being.

When the final state of meditation is reached and the soul is isolated, it automatically becomes a part of *Puruṣa.* Binding of the individual soul with the cycle of birth and death is due to the remains of *karma* called *saṃskāra* and as soon as the freedom from these are obtained, there is no identity of the individual soul and it joins the indestructible and unbound eternal cosmic energy. This is the aim of Patañjali's yoga.

PRACTICE OF YOGA (PART II)

The Part II of the *Yogasūtra* is about the details of the practical aspects and techniques. The practice of yoga involves austerity, silent repetition of a mantra and a profound devotion to *Īśvara* or the Absolute. Austerity is to reduce the actions, which give rise to sensuous pleasure. This leads one to have control over one's senses and mind. Silent repetition of a mantra gives rise to steadiness of the mind. Devotion to *Īśvara* is the devotion to the cause of yoga. It is to submit oneself to the aim and to get rid of one's identity associated to one's physical self.

Kleśa or the afflictions

The purpose of the above said three major practices is to extenuate the afflictions or *kleśa.* The *kleśas* are ignorance, egotism, desire, aversion and attachment. The base of all *kleśas* is *avidyā* or ignorance and that is to consider the non-eternal and distressful material reality as eternal and joyful. Because of the ephemeral nature of the worldly things and even the joys and pleasures of the world ultimately drag us into pain.

Identity of oneself with one's physical being is egotism.

Desire or *rāga* is a longing and thirst for enjoyment. It makes one's mind slave to the senses and thus is antagonist for obtaining the concentration of the mind.

Aversion or *dveṣa* is the feeling that arises out of distress and is usually directed against something or someone.

Attachment or *abhiniveśa* is an inherent quality in all living beings to remain alive. It is the attachment to our physical self and the fear of pain and death.

There are four different forms of afflictions:

1. Dormant afflictions are awakened in mind by certain associations related to those experiences.
2. Extenuated afflictions are subdued through meditation.
3. Intercepted afflictions are those, which are overpowered by certain antagonistic afflictions, like desire is overpowered by aversion.
4. Overt afflictions are expressed when their causative agent is present

Liberation from *kleśa*

Subtle afflictions like *abhiniveśa* or tenacity to life may give rise to fear of death, pain, insecurity and so on. They should be evaded by antagonist ideas like recognising the real self, soul and detaching oneself from the ephemeral body.

Gross afflictions like desire (*rāga*) and aversion (*dveṣa*) should be got rid by a continuous intentness of the mind.

The stock of the previous *karma* is the base of afflictions and at birth the afflictions may be visible or hidden. That means that the accumulated *karma* from previous life or lives may unfold themselves at birth or later as the occasions come. The *karma* unfold themselves at an appropriate occasion as they are related to other people and places. At a right time, space and opportunity, our give and take or other kinds of exchange with others take place. This, however, does not mean that everything is determined before hand. The present *karma* intervenes and thus the joys and sorrows we experience in life are the combination of the result of previous and the present *karma.* In other words, we have to go through the results of our previous *karma,* but how we handle the existing circumstances with our present *karma* can make a tremendous difference. For example, if we are rich due to our past *karma,* how we manage with the wealth will decide about many of the future events. If we do good deeds like donation, helping the poor and the needy and other acts of this kind, we further accumulate good *karma* and due to that, we may gain more wealth. In a similar case, we may not do good deeds but invest the wealth intelligently and also gain more wealth in this case. But it is quite possible that the stock of our good *karma* may get exhausted one day and we may suffer not necessarily the financial loss but in other ways like from an ailment, emotional disturbances and so on. As has been said in Section I, we ourselves are responsible for doing good or bad *karma,* and that we choose with our ability to discriminate, the *buddhi. Buddhi* is the *sattva* state of mind. With yogic practices, we can reach a level of mental lucidity and at that state our actions and decisions are driven by *buddhi,* and not heart or mind. Thus, attaining a lucid state of mind is essential and beneficial not only for a yogī but also for a normal worldly person for attaining emotional and spiritual strength and for the well-being of present and future.

Patañjali affirms that 'while there is the root (of the deeds in afflictions), they bear fruits (in the form of) birth, age and experience. These depending upon virtuous and non-virtuous deeds, lead to enjoyable and painful fruits' (Part II, Sūtra 13,14). That means the conditions of birth and its circumstances are determined by our previous *karma.* But a wise person should understand that what appears enjoyable is also ultimately painful. It means that because of the transitory nature of everything in this world, nothing stays forever and departure of joy leads ultimately to pain. Therefore, if we keep equilibrium during happy times, we do not suffer from pain when the happiness or joy is no more there. It means that one should avoid the pain that is not yet there.

The conjunction of the 'onlooker' with the 'scene' should be abandoned. The onlooker is the soul and the scene is the phenomenal world, which is being looked at by the intellect. The soul is not bound to action whereas the intellect is the attribute of the three principal qualities or *guṇas* (*sattva, rajas* and *tamas*) which bind us to action or *karma.* The soul passively observes the activities of the mind but it is without qualities and is not involved with the phenomenal world. However, it is the cause of all knowledge as it is the light that makes the seeing possible. It is the soul, which is truly experiencing yet it is not involved with the experience, as it is not undergoing modifications. It is always still. When the vision of the phenomenal world stops for one particular person, this vision does not cease to be and it is there for other persons. The phenomenal world continues to be as usual for other individuals. Thus, there is diversity of the Cosmic Substance, *Prakṛti,* whereas there is non-diversity of the Universal Soul, *Puruṣa.*

With the above-said conjunction, one is unable to differentiate the power that sees (soul) from the power that simply cognises the sensuous experience. For the wise, these two powers remain distinctly different. The cause of conjunction between the two different and distinct powers is ignorance or *avidyā.* Thus, if we have the wisdom to realise that soul is the cause of our being and our real self, it is distinct from the senses and the mind and is the ultimate energy and truth, we will not have afflictions or *kleśa.* By the absence of above-said conjunction, there is total isolation of the soul or *kaivalya.*

Kaivalya is the aim of the *Yogasūtra of Patañjali.* Once the soul is isolated, it is no more bound to *karma* and *saṃsāra* (the cycle of life and death). Soul is a part of the *Puruṣa* or the Absolute and when it has no *karmic* binding left, it gets dissolved in the Absolute.

Continuous presence of *viveka* or the discriminative knowledge about *Puruṣa* and *Prakṛti* being distinct from each other destroys the above-said conjunction. This conjunction forms a bridge between the soul and the world. When it is destroyed, the soul remains uninvolved with the world.

Aṣṭāṅga Yoga or the eight-fold yogic practice

It is important to destroy afflictions or *kleśa* to obtain *viveka* or the discriminative knowledge and that is done through various yogic practices. There are eight yogic practices described by Patañjali and these are known as Patañjali's *Aṣṭāṅga Yoga* (the eight-fold yogic practice). I am giving these practices in Table 5 which is reproduced from my book on the *Yogasūtra* for a quick glance[5]. We will discuss each of these steps in detail in following page. The first five practices are described in this Part and the rest three are in Part III.

The eight different parts of the yogic practices are like the steps of a ladder. Each is independent and makes a base for the next step. Each accomplished step takes us a degree higher towards the goal.

The first of the eight practices is called *yama* or restraint. There are five *yamas.* The first is not to kill or cause pain to others. It is called *ahiṃsā.* Directly or indirectly harming others or causing pain or motivating others for such acts come in this category. *Ahiṃsā* was preached intensively by many saints of ancient India during this period when *Yogasūtras* were written (6th and 7th century BC) and the most prominent amongst them are Gautama Buddha and Lord Mahāvīra. The followers of these saints founded later on the two major religions, Buddhism and Jainism. They, particularly the Jainas follow the tradition of *ahiṃsā* very strictly still today. Earlier, India was largely a meat-eating country, and the Buddha and Mahāvīra had influenced greatly the living tradition and that is why India remains until today a largely vegetarian country.

It is interesting to note that the largely meat-eating West has recently been influenced by the yogic culture of *ahiṃsā* and there have been movements of vegetarianism. Besides that, there is an awakening in people about not killing and paining animals. There are groups who are fighting against killing animals for their leather and fur goods, hunting and against many other actions that involve *hiṃsā* (violence, killing and paining). However, there is another category of people who will participate in all these demonstrations of cruelty against animals, will take care of the smallest insect but they are meat eaters. My discussions with such people in several Western countries reveal that they do not

---

5 V. Verma, The *Yogasūtra of Patañjali: A Scientific Exposition,* 1996, Clarion Books, New Delhi, India

Table 5. A summary of the eight-fold path of yogic practice or *Aṣṭāṅga Yoga.*

1. Forbearance or *yama*	A. *Ahiṃsā:* or not killing or paining others
	B. *Satya:* veracity or truthfulness
	C. *Asteya:* not stealing
	D. *Brahmacarya:* continence, i.e., self-restraint from yielding to impulse or desire
	E. *Aparigraha:* not coveting, i.e., not desiring for oneself the means of enjoyment.
2. Self-discipline or *niyama*	A. *Śauca:* purification — Physical; Mental
	B. *Santoṣa:* contentment
	C. *Tapa:* austerity
	D. *Jāpa:* silent repetition of a mantra
	E. *Īśvarapraṇidhāna:* a profound devotion to the *Īśvara* (*Puruṣa*).
3. Yogic postures or *āsana*	The special postures devised for the purpose of yoga. They should become steady and pleasant with continuous practice.
4. *Prāṇāyāma*	*Prāṇāyāma* is the expansion of vital energy. Its practice involves a progressive deceleration of the respiratory rhythm and increasing the intervals between inhaling and exhaling and vice versa.
5. Restraint or *pratyāhāra*	*Pratyāhāra* is the indifference of the senses to their objects and their uniformity with the nature of the mind. Objects of senses are colour for sight and sound for hearing etc.
6. *Dhāraṇā* (attention)	*Dhāraṇā* is fixing the thinking principle on internal space (*deśa*).
7. *Dhyāna* (contemplation)	*Dhyānā* is a continuous state of *dhāraṇā.*
8. *Samādhi* (meditation)	*Samādhi* is when *dhyānā* reaches a state where only the awareness of its meaning remains and even the personal identity is lost.

Note: It is not possible to find the exact equivalent in English for the last three yogic practices. However, the tentative translation has been given in parenthesis.

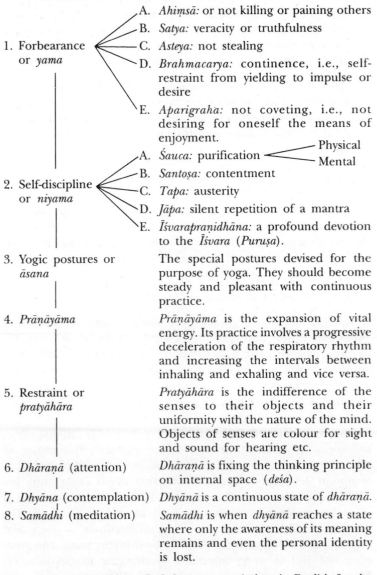

consider meat eating against *ahiṃsā* as they are not involved in killing. Indeed, it is a paradoxical attitude and it amounts to not owning the responsibility for one's deeds. But in the present context of Patañjali's yoga, they are committing an act of hiṃsā as much as if they killed the animals themselves. In Sūtra 34 of this Part, Patañjali says very specifically:

> **'Questionable acts such as killing etc., whether done, caused to be done or approved of, whether resulting from greed, anger or attachment, whether slight, intermediate or beyond measure, result in endless pain and destroy wisdom; hence should be opposed.'**

The second *yama* is to always speak the truth and never to distort it or tell lies. The third *yama* is not to steel or take away things from others. The fourth *yama* is continence, which means to exercise restraint on yielding to impulse or desire or any of the bodily activities. Not to covet is the fifth *yama*, which means not to desire for oneself the means of enjoyment.

> **'These (*yamas*), irrespective of caste, place, period, time, are the great universal duties' (Sūtra 31).**

Patañjali is very categorical here about *ahiṃsā* and the other *yamas* and affirms that one cannot say that someone is a butcher by profession or caste and therefore is exempt from killing or another person is a medical student or researcher and may be liberated from this duty. Or under certain circumstances or at certain places or at certain age, one can eat meat or tell lies or steal and so on.

The second of the eight-fold yogic practices is self-discipline, which consists of 1) purification, 2) contentment, 3) austerity, 4) silent repetition of a mantra or a sound or a symbol and 5) a profound devotion to *Īśvara*. Purification needs explanation because it is physical as well as mental. The physical purification is done by cleaning the body externally as well as internally. For internal purification, there are several methods in yoga like cleaning the nasal passage, cleaning by drinking water and vomiting out and cleaning intestines by drinking excessive water. Mental purification means to get rid of afflictions.

When the adept of yoga has developed an attitude of complete harmlessness towards the creatures around him/her, even the dangerous and aggressive animals do not attack and are in harmony with him/her.

The adept who practises complete veracity gets the fruits of good deeds even without performing those deeds.

The abstinence from theft gives rise to an expression of complete trustworthiness and the adept gets many precious offerings.

When continence is complete, strength and vigour are gained.

Covetousness is not merely the means of enjoyment but it is also soul's coveting of the body.

Purification gives rise to censoring one's own body and in that case, no desire is left for another person's body. In addition to that, purification leads to subjugation of senses and intentness of mind.[6]

The second part of self-discipline is contentment or *santoṣa.* This gives rise to inner joy. The third part of self-discipline or *niyama* is austerity, which gradually leads to the removal of afflictions, and thereafter the senses attain a higher discerning power.

Japa or the silent repetition of a mantra leads to the vision of one's favourite deity or of whatever the mantra is aimed at. The perfection in meditation comes from profound devotion to *Īśvara.* However, if *japa* is done with mantra OṂ and with devotion, it leads to perfection. We have already discussed above that Patañjali refers to *Puruṣa* or the Absolute by the word *Īśvara.*

Third of the eight yogic practices is *āsana* or a yogic posture. Patañjali defines it as that 'which is steady and pleasant'. That means that when one is in a particular yogic posture, it should be as comfortable as normal sitting posture and then only we can say that *āsana* has achieved perfection. There should be no wavering or trembling and one should not feel unpleasant or uncomfortable while in an *āsana.* This is achieved by gradual practice and concentration. The extent of effort one has to make depends upon an individual's body flexibility and health conditions. *Āsana* is to enhance the steadiness of the body and that

---

[6] Many Hindus worship ritualistically (*pūjā*) every morning and it is customary to do that immediately after bath. It is advised not to be interrupted between bath and *pūjā.* Similarly, before the bath, it is considered very important to evacuate and clean one's tongue and throat properly. Even this minor form of purification leads to better concentration during *pūjā.*

leads to the steadiness of the mind. After having achieved mastery on *āsana*, one is not affected by extreme conditions like cold, heat, hunger, thirst and so on.

The fourth of the eight yogic practices is *prāṇāyāma*, which should be practised after the *āsana*. It is a regulated inhalation and exhalation with intervals. The three aspects of *prāṇāyāma* are long or short and are directed by place, time and number. The outer (*bāhya*) refers to exhalation, the inner (*ābhyantara*) refers to inhalation and the steady (*stambha*) refers to when one is holding the breath inside or holding the lungs without air. These three terms originally used by Patañjali are later referred to as *recaka, pūraka* and *kumbhaka* respectively. These three are more popular in modern day yoga terminology.

The outer and inner and the steady are directed by place, time and number and then termed as long or short. The place refers to the part of the body to which vital air is guided. The time is the duration of performance and the number refers to the number of repetitions of the process of inhalation, exhalation and the steady state.

The fourth aspect of *prāṇāyāma* assumes 'both the outer and the inner spheres' (Sūtra 51). After practising *prāṇāyāma* for a long period, the inhalation and exhalation are reduced to such a degree that the restraint of breath is spontaneously achieved. The transfer from motion to steady state is no longer sudden.

The soul is the pure form of wisdom. It is that light or energy which puts life into the material body. However, we are unable to use this Inner Light as it is covered with the darkness of *avidyā* or ignorance. The ignorance is to mistake our physical self as our real self and eternal. *Avidyā* forms a thick and dark blanket, which obstruct the light emerging from our inner source, soul. Practice of *prāṇāyāma* weakens this obstruction of the Inner Light. That means, it destroys *avidyā*.

With the removal of *avidyā*, the mind becomes capable of attention or *dhāraṇā*, which is sixth of the eight yogic practices.

The fifth of the eight yogic stages is or *pratyāhāra*. It is the indifference of the senses to their objects and their uniformity with the nature of the mind. Object of sight is form and colour, object of hearing is sound and so on. When senses abandon their objects and abide in their own nature, then the mind acquires complete control over the senses and becomes capable of controlling them. In other words, we withdraw the senses temporarily from their capabilities and control their functions with our will. This is called the subjugation of senses.

THE ACCOMPLISHMENTS OF YOGA (PART III)

The last three of the eight yogic practices are described in the beginning of Part III. These are *dhāraṇā, dhyāna* and *samādhi.*

Dhāraṇā may be translated as attention or concentration. It is defined as 'Fixing the thinking principle on the internal space' (Sūtra 1). The internal space means the energy points of the body like areas around the navel, around the plexus, between the eyes, tip of the tongue etc. Later, in the history of yoga, different energy points acquired very sophisticated nomenclature and were called the seven *cakras* or the concentric energy points of the subtle body. The *Yoga Upaniṣad* also mentions the *cakras*[7]. However, it is very difficult to mention the chronological order of this evolution. (See Section I, Figure 6 for the details of the *cakras*).

A continuum of *dhāraṇā* is *dhyāna. Dhāraṇā* can be compared to continuous drops of falling water whereas *dhyāna* is like the flow of a liquid of thick consistency like oil.

Samādhi is the last of the eight yogic practices and is defined as when *dhyāna* reaches a state where only awareness of its meaning remains and even the personal identity is lost. That means when *dhyāna* reaches a state when only the consciousness of its aim remains and other consciousness is lost, it is termed as *samādhi* or meditation. This is a state where consciousness of the fact that 'I am meditating' is also lost.

A continuous practice of *samādhi* will give rise to the state of *saṃyama* (mastery over oneself) and that ultimately gives rise to a discerning ability. Discerning ability is beyond the normal worldly abilities and it is the capacity to detect which is small, hidden and far away.

The discerning ability gives rise to new modifications of the mind. Then *saṃyama* should be used (*viniyoga*) again to stop these new modifications.

In Sūtra 7 of this Part, Patañjali states that *dhāraṇā, dhyāna* and *samādhi* are distinct from the previously described five yogic practices. The earlier five practices (*yama, niyama* etc.) are pre-

---

[7] *Yoga Upaniṣad,* IV, 2-20

paratory to these three, *dhāraṇā, dhyāna* and *samādhi.* And these three are preparatory to the meditation without seed.

The state of mind resulting from *samādhi* is denoted by the rise of intentness on a single point (*ekāgratā*) and fall of diverted attention (dissolution of multiple diversions of attention). By repeated practice, the adept of yoga develops the *saṃskāra* of *samādhi.* That means that the previous *saṃskāra* of the adept gradually vanish and instead the *saṃskāra* of *samādhi* develops. At this stage, the adept is capable of achieving various special powers or accomplishments called *siddhis* by doing *saṃyama* on specific objects and concepts.

Siddhis

Siddhis are interpreted as supernatural powers in some yoga texts. You may have heard about yogīs capable of doing very unusual things like walking on water or disappearing or having ability to see things which normal human beings cannot see. Technically, these capabilities are called *siddhis,* which are the accomplishment of the constant meditative practices. Following is the description of various *siddhis,* which are attained by performing *saṃyama*:

1. The first *siddhi* described by Patañjali is the attainment of the knowledge of past and future, which is achieved by performing *saṃyama* on the three fold modifications of diverse objects and subjects.
   The three fold modifications are the three states of modifications of the five elements. These three states are: A. Characteristics (*dharma*), which is the principal characteristic and the characterised matter is called *dharmī.* B. Symptom (*lakṣaṇa*) is the material manifestation of that matter. C. Condition (*avasthā*) is the state of that matter which is subjected to time. To understand these three states, the famous example of a clay pitcher or a jar is given in the yogic texts. A jar is made out of a lump of clay. The clay assumes another shape than its lumpiness when it is moulded into a jar. The characterised substance, which is earth, is termed as *dharmī.* The symptom is in the form of indication that the jar existed already in the clay and it only became visible when the potter removed the superfluous parts from it. The jar in present form represents the present

whereas after being destroyed, it becomes a part of the clay again and thus becomes a part of the past. The jar is constantly undergoing modifications.

By performing *saṃyama* on the three states of diverse objects, a yogī is able to attain the knowledge about its past and future. For example, if a yogī performs *saṃyama* on a table and the three states of modifications, he can know from where the wood for the table came, where the tree was grown and when the table will come to an end or degenerate and so on.

2. A yogī can attain the capability of comprehending the speeches of all living beings by performing *saṃyama* on the division of word, meaning and the sense attached to it. Normally, we see a word, its meaning and the sense attached to it as one. For example, when we perceive a tree, we see as the word 'tree' identical to the notion this word arises in our mind due to previous knowledge and the reality of the tree with its roots, stem, foliage etc. These three are separate entities and a yogī is capable of comprehending this. Thus, by performing *saṃyama* on these three, a yogī gets the second *siddhi* to comprehend the speeches of all the animals and different languages spoken by human beings.
3. *Saṃskāra* are the remains of our past deeds. By performing *saṃyama* on these, a yogī is capable of comprehending their origin from the past lives. That means he or she will be able to visualise when and how and due to which deeds they were accumulated.
4. When the adept of yoga performs *saṃyama* on the knowledge of some characteristics of the other person like the appearance, he or she attains the *siddhi* of knowing the mind of that particular person. However, this *siddhi* has its limitation, as the adept cannot know what the intentions of the other persons are as these are external to the nature of the mind.
5. When the adept performs *saṃyama* on the form of his/her own body, the perceivable power of that form vanishes. That means that the others are incapable of perceiving the body of the adept. The adept acquires the capability of disappearing for others while he or she is still present.

6. The adept acquires the *siddhi* of foreseeing the end of his/her physical self by performing *saṃyama* on the two-fold *karma.* The two-fold *karma* are the ones which fructify quickly and the ones which fructify after a long period of time.
7. By friendship, compassion etc., towards all (good, bad, friendly, unfriendly human beings)., the adept acquires the immense inner power.
8. When the adept performs *saṃyama* on the physical strength, he or she acquires the power similar to that of an elephant.
9. By performing *saṃyama* on the sensuous cognition, the adept acquires the *siddhi* to see the minute, the concealed and the distant objects.
10. By performing *saṃyama* on the sun, the adept acquires the knowledge of the universe. In the body, the point above the plexus is symbolic of sun and the *saṃyama* is performed on this energy point.
11. The *siddhi* to attain knowledge about the star arrangement comes to the adept by performing *saṃyama* on the moon. The tip of the nose is said to be the symbol of moon in yogic literature[8]. Thus, the yogī acquires knowledge of star constellation by performing *saṃyama* on this symbolic point for the moon.
12. Further on, the knowledge about the movements of the stars is attained by performing *saṃyama* on the polar star. In this case, there is no point of the body, which symbolises the polar star.
13. By performing *saṃyama* on the circle of the navel, the adept acquires the knowledge of the bodily systems. The circle around the navel is considered to be the principal meridian from where all the other parts originate. That means, the three humours (*vāta, pitta* and *kapha*) and the seven materials or *dhātus* (skin, bones, flesh, nerves, blood, bone marrow and semen) originate from the area around the navel.[9]
14. The adept of yoga can get over the feeling of thirst and hunger by performing *saṃyama* on the deeper part of the throat or the pit of the throat.

---

[8] *Gheraṇḍa Saṃhitā*, V, 43.

[9] The circle around the navel is a very important energy point for healing various ailments. The practical aspect of these healing practices will be taken up later in the book.

15. By performing *saṃyama* below the pit of the throat (opening of the bronchial tube), the adept attains stability. That means that he or she can stay a long time without moving, just like the hibernating animals.
16. In the centre of the skull, there is an aperture, which is an energy point of the subtle body and it is called the cerebral light. By performing *saṃyama* on this point, the adept can have a vision of all those yogīs who have attained *siddhis* in the past.
17. By performing *saṃyama* on the area around the heart, the adept acquires the knowledge of his or her own mind and of the minds of the other persons. The area around the heart is the symbolic meeting point of the body and the soul.
18. By breaking the bondage between the body and the mind, the adept acquires the *siddhi* to enter into other persons' bodies. The identification of the body and the mind has to be severed by the adept to acquire this power.
19. The mastery of the practice of *prāṇāyāma*, which is called *udāna* (conducting the vital air upward to the head), the adept develops the capacity to rise above deep water or thick mud and remains unaffected by thorns.
20. *Samāna* is that when the vital air is conducted towards the navel region and by the mastery over this practice of the *prāṇāyāma*, the adept acquires a radiant look.
21. The adept develops a divine power of hearing by performing *saṃyama* on the sense of hearing and ether. Ether is the medium of all what we hear. Our capacity for hearing is limited because it is distance-dependent. By performing *saṃyama* between these two factors, the adept is capable of hearing subtle and distant sounds.
22. The adept acquires the power of moving in ether by obtaining a state of lightness like cotton by performing *saṃyama* on the relationship of the body to the ether. That means that the adept is able to detach from the other four elements the body is made of and he wins over the ether or space to be able to move around freely.
23. By performing *saṃyama* on the five fundamental elements (ether, air, fire, water and earth) and their qualities, the

adept attains the eight great *siddhis*. These are:

a. acquiring a minute structure of the body,
b. capability of magnifying oneself,
c. capability of becoming heavy,
d. capability of becoming almost weightless,
e. power of touching distant objects,
f. power to get into the earth and come back,
g. power to subjugate the objects, and
h. creative power of command on the elements.

After attainment of these eight *siddhis*, the adept reaches perfection and cannot be affected by fire, water, wind etc. He or she acquires beauty, charm, strength and adamantine power.

After having described all the *siddhis*, Patañjali tells us that there is also an alternative way to attain these *siddhis*, which is by attaining the knowledge about the ultimate truth, the *Puruṣa* or the cause of being of the phenomenal world. The realisation of this ultimate truth leads to a higher form of knowledge about the subtle, concealed and distant things.

The *siddhis* and the aim of yoga

Siddhis are the achievements of meditation but they are not the goal of the yoga of Patañjali. Patañjali warns that the *siddhis* or the special accomplishments of meditation may become obstacle for an adept. If the adept displays the *siddhis* to others and their appreciation may give rise to egotism in the adept and he or she may return to the worldly pleasures again. The special accomplishments should be used to conquer sense organs. After having conquered the sense organs, the adept acquires a mind-like rapidity in his/her body motions and becomes capable of getting the sense organ function independent of the body. The adept also attains the capability of altering things from one state to another.

The adept must remain indifferent to his accomplishments and state of perfection, and this will destroy the germ of perniciousness. When this latter is achieved, the yogī succeeds in attaining the state of *kaivalya* or total isolation. The soul is totally isolated from the body made of five elements and three qualities. This is the ultimate goal of the yoga as when the soul is totally isolated, it becomes a part of the *Puruṣa* or the Universal Soul and the yogi gets rid of the cycle of birth and death and attains eternality.

THE ABSOLUTE ISOLATION OR *KAIVALYA* (PART IV)

The fourth Part of the *Yogasūtra* deals with the profound philosophical and logical analysis of the concepts used in the previous three Parts.

Patañjali begins the last Part of his book by revealing that there are also other means of obtaining *siddhis* than meditation. Some people have specific gifts from birth. These are due to their previous *saṃskāra. Siddhis* may also be obtained for a limited period of time by taking some narcotic drugs. The third means to attain *siddhis* is by repetition of mantras. The fourth means of obtaining *siddhis* is by austere practices that strengthen the mind and enable one to attain extraordinary mental powers.

However, *siddhis,* which are obtained by meditation have a different aim. They should be used to conquer the senses and to detach oneself from the world. These *siddhis,* unlike the others are different because they are for the aim of yoga, which is total isolation or *kaivalya.* The *siddhis* obtained by other means described above may also be used for the purpose of yoga by fulfilling other conditions, like *yama, niyama* etc., which are prescribed for an adept of yoga in the eight-fold yogic practices.

Some people have *siddhis* like healing others or knowing the other persons' mind or capability of knowing about the past lives or about the happenings of the future and so on. In many instances, these *siddhis* are congenital. Generally these are used for the worldly purpose like displaying them for fame, admiration and money or for a social cause like healing. Some people mistake these category of persons with yogīs, which is a false notion. However, these fundamental capabilities can be altered in their purpose for the aim of the yoga, which is to attain a total isolation of the soul from all what belongs to the phenomenal world.

A yogīs has the capability of creating numerous bodies and minds only after he/she has achieved the aim of the yoga. These created minds are without afflictions and without *saṃskāra.* It is the mind of the yogī, which is the principal governing force for these created minds.

Patañjali has written about the three-fold division of *karma,* which is essentially based upon the three principal *guṇas* of the

Prakṛti. These are the following:

1. Vicious, evil, wicked *karma,* which do harm to others are called *kṛṣṇa karma* (black deeds).
2. Those actions, which are associated with virtue like giving alms, leading an austere life, doing selfless work for the good of others are called *śukla karma* (white deeds).
3. *Śukla-kṛṣṇa karma* are the combination of the two types of deeds described above. The deeds done by most of us in our day-to-day existence generally fall in this category. For example, a farmer while ploughing his fields may kill small insects. In certain situations, we may be obliged to tell lies.

The *karma* of a yogī do not belong to any of these three categories. They are neutral. That means that they do not build further new *saṃskāra.* After having achieved *kaivalya,* a *yogī* is no more involved in the phenomenal world. The element of *Puruṣa* in him/her is isolated from *prakṛti* and the yogī is no more bound by any actions.

The three types of *karma* described above give rise to results, which in turn give rise to the fruits of those actions in the form of pain and pleasure. The experience of pain and pleasure is called *vāsanā.* In other words, the three types of deeds or *karma* lead us to further deeds as we enjoy or suffer their fruits and remain bound to further action.

All our experiences are stored in the form of memory in our minds. Due to change of place or large time interval, we may think that we have forgotten certain events, but on an appropriate occasion and through various associations, all the previous experiences are recalled. *Saṃskāra* or the remains of previous *karma* have a quality similar to memory, but in this case the time span is longer than one life span. The results of *karma* may be intercepted for a certain period of time but they reappear at an appropriate occasion. For example, if someone has *saṃskāra* of a scholar from previous life, they may not appear immediately after birth due to the opposing circumstances. The opposing circumstances may be like birth in a family where there is no intellectual atmosphere. However, when this child goes to school, he or she spontaneously gets attracted to learning and to scholarly teachers. It is easier to understand this if we think that *saṃskāra* are like memory but over a longer period of time. The past experiences reappear in a subtle form.

Tenacity to life is an innate quality in all living beings. Instinct for eternity originates from *ahaṃkāra* or the individuating principle, which gives rise to identity and attachment to life. Even in the smallest of living beings, the love for life and instinct for eternity is observed.

The fundamental cause of the experience of pleasure and pain (*vāsanā*) is ignorance or *avidyā*, which is due to inability to realise the non-eternal character of the worldly things. *Vāsanā* gives rise to further action and the substratum of *karma* is accumulated in the form of *saṃskāra*. Desires and aim for seeking fruits of actions provide support to *vāsanā*. This is due to *avidyā* from which further *karma* and *saṃskāra* originate. These four; the cause, the effect, the substratum and the support form a wheel of the worldly existence. This idea is illustrated in Table 6.[10]

Whatever exists has a nature of its own and cannot assume a state of non-entity. All existing things modify according to their three-fold nature (the three *guṇas*). With the passing time, the things undergo modification and acquire an altered state. With this statement, Patañjali wishes to emphasise that the above-described cycle of cause, effect, substratum and support is in the form of altered state and removal of the cause of accumulation of *saṃskāra* does not imply the non-entity of the existence.

The three qualities exist in the manifest and the subtle but there is a variation in the ratio of these three qualities, which is responsible for the individual attributes of their properties. One thing differs from another because of the variations in the degree of each *guṇa*. The unity in the essential nature of all objects is due to the fact that they all have three fundamental qualities of the Cosmic Substance and they all undergo constant modifications.

An object and its perception by the mind are two distinct entities. The same object may appear different or evoke different feelings in different individuals. The perception and the thought about an object are not the reality of an object. They both remain distinct from each other due to the diversity in individual minds and thought processes. A hunted animal for a meat eater may

---

[10] This table is from my book *The Yogasūtras of Patañjali: A Scientific Exposition*, 1996, Clarion Books, New Delhi.

give rise to a feeling of joy and evoke appetite whereas for an animal lover or an adept of yoga, it may evoke disgust for the killer and compassion for the animal.

Tabel 6. An illustration of the four factors (the cause, the effect, the substratum and the support) which together form an eternal cycle of *vāsanā, saṃskāra* and *karma* leading to an endless cycle of birth and death (*saṃsāra*).

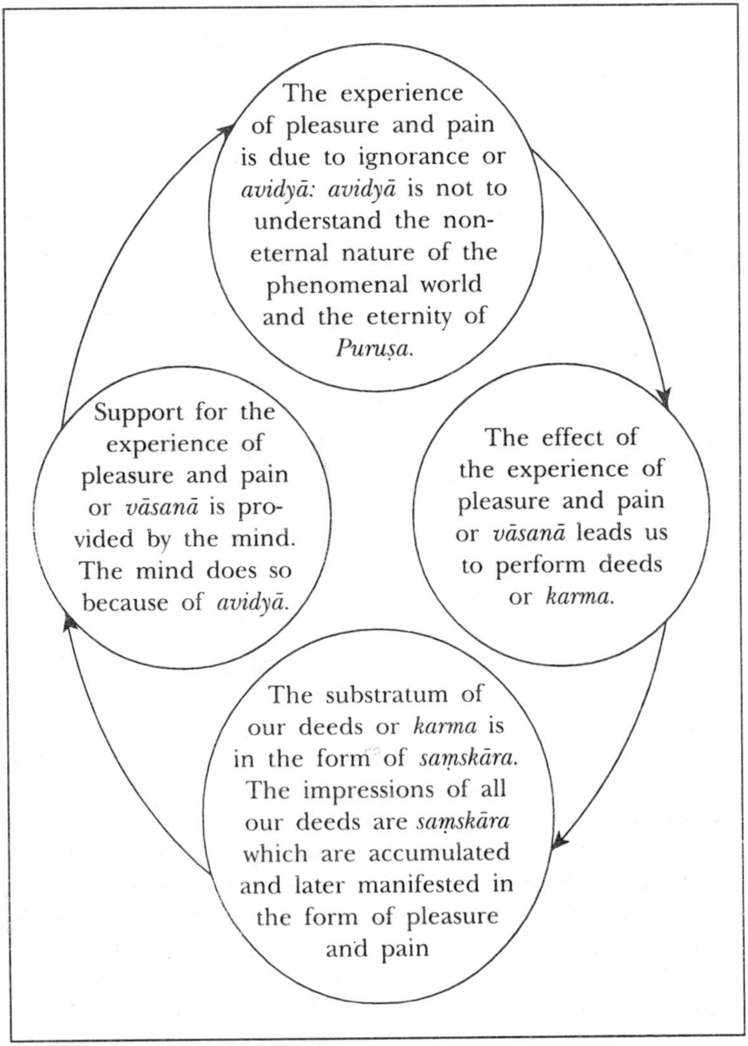
The experience of pleasure and pain is due to ignorance or avidyā: avidyā is not to understand the non-eternal nature of the phenomenal world and the eternity of Puruṣa.
The effect of the experience of pleasure and pain or vāsanā leads us to perform deeds or karma.
The substratum of our deeds or karma is in the form of saṃskāra. The impressions of all our deeds are saṃskāra which are accumulated and later manifested in the form of pleasure and pain
Support for the experience of pleasure and pain or vāsanā is provided by the mind. The mind does so because of avidyā.

Further, Patañjali says that the reality of an object is not dependent upon the conception of a single mind as in that case what an object would be without knowledge? If it were so, then in case of lack of conception about that object, it will become non-existent. Thus, an object has its existence independent of any conception regarding it. For example, if we fall down while walking because of a ditch in the path, it is our lack of knowledge about that ditch, which became a hindrance for us. The ditch that caused the fall existed even though we did not know about it. Thus, the reality of an object is independent of any conception about that particular object.

An object attracts the mind like a magnet attracts a piece of iron. It becomes known to the mind through the sense organs and is cognised by the intellect. The objects, which do not become apparent to the mind are not cognised and remain unknown to it. The mind constantly undergoes modifications and its modifications are always known to the soul, as that does not undergo modifications. If it were also undergoing modifications, then it would not have been possible that all the modifications of the mind become known to it. Then there would have been two different sorts of modifications independent of each other. For example, a number of turning wheels, when reflected in a still mirror can be distinctly seen to be turning. However, if we start to turn the mirror also, we will not be able to get the information about the turning wheels. There will be a confusion of the reflected images of the turning wheels in the turning mirror.

The mind is perceived by the soul and that is why it is not self-illuminating. The soul is not further perceived by anything else and is self-illuminating. The mind identifies itself with the feelings of pleasure, pain, anger etc., it is not a mere perceiver of all these emotions. If we are able to control the modifications of the mind and severe its sensuous identity until it is merely an uninvolved onlooker, it identifies itself with the self-illuminating soul.

The mind cannot ascertain the knowledge and the consciousness of knowing at the same time. The moment of perception cannot be simultaneously the moment of realisation that I am the perceiver.

If we consider the oneness of the soul and the mind and then within one mind various minds and intellects so that cognition by one mind is further cognised by another, then there would be confusion. In other words, in this case, it would not be the soul, which is the perceiver, but another mind and another intellect. Patañjali invalidates this concept by saying that in this situation, a confusion of memory will occur because one notion would be needed to illuminate another and that there would be a necessity of endless notions. Similarly, to recollect a particular notion, many notions may be produced simultaneously causing a confusion of memory.

Self-realisation of an object perceived takes place only when the mind as perceiver has the notion of an object that does not change any further and this immutable mental power relating to that object comes in contact with the intellect (*buddhi*). The *buddhi* is the *sattva* element of the mind. Immutable mental power related to an object is that when the three qualities related to that perception do not change any more.

The thinking principle of the mind (*citta*) is omniscient, as it perceives both soul and the object to be perceived. On one hand, the mind is attracted to the worldly objects like a magnet to a piece of iron, on the other hand, it is only through the mind that the realisation of *Puruṣa* is achieved. That is why, the mind is omniscient. Despite being the site of innumerable experiences, the mind does not have its independent existence as it can only operate in association with the soul. The mind is incapable of having the consciousness of the experiences without the association of the soul.

The individuating principle is one of the three components that result from the association of *Puruṣa* and *Prakṛti*. It gives rise to feeling of identity in a being. By getting rid of it, one becomes capable of seeing different notions in their purity, instead of experiencing them with involvement. This experience of purity of perception gives rise to *viveka* or the discriminative knowledge that enables the adept to distinguish between *Puruṣa* and *Prakṛti* and thus, leads to *kaivalya* or the total isolation of the soul.

The *saṃskāra* are not destroyed immediately after attaining the discriminative knowledge. They are weakened but are nevertheless revived in mind from time to time. By a continuous presence of the discriminative knowledge, *saṃskāra* are diminished and gradually, they totally vanish. When the adept remains completely uninvolved with this achievement, then arise the complete discriminative knowledge or *dharmamegha samādhi*. This is a state when *karma* and *saṃskāra* are completely terminated. The yogi is no longer bound or compelled to further action or to the cycle of birth and death. The cycle of birth and death is due to previous *karma*. At this state, the yogī has achieved absolute freedom and has no bondage with his/her body. The three qualities of *prakṛti* do not exist for a yogī and neither the modifications related to each moment of time.

The complete dissolution of the qualities in reference to the soul of the yogī or the power of mind in its own nature is *kaivalya*. The qualities are terminated for that particular soul of the yogī and not for the cosmos as such. The soul, which is a part of the Universal Soul or *Puruṣa* is without any qualities and gets involved with the qualities of the Cosmic Substance or *prakṛti* when in association with it. The total isolation or *kaivalya* dissociates this binding of *Puruṣa* and *Prakṛti*, which is in the form of soul and body in an individual and he or she gets the eternal freedom from the bondage with the phenomenal world. At this state, the power of the mind is in its own nature. That means that it is dissociated from the phenomenal world and reflects the nature of the soul. As said earlier, the mind perceives the object as well as the soul. The mind of the yogī uninvolved with the world due to discriminative knowledge, reflects the nature of the soul.

SECTION III
Fundamentals of Āyurveda

Āyurveda is the wisdom about life from ancient India. Some call it science of life. Āyurveda tells us the art of living and when there are hindrances like mental or physical pain, disorders, ailments and diseases, it provides remedies for those and prescribes methods to bring the body to equilibrium and harmony again. Āyurveda also includes the science of rejuvenation in order to enhance vitality and minimise the effect of aging. Āyurveda is not merely the medical system from ancient India as is understood by many. It is a comprehensive science of life which also provides you suggestions about how to live an enriched, happy and disease-free life and how to enhance the pleasures of life. It also instructs on optimising the quality of life and enhancing life span. All this is done not only with remedies of natural origin and balanced nutrition but also with your mental and spiritual efforts. The word '*Āyuḥ*' in fact means age (the time between birth and death) and Veda means wisdom. Thus, this scriptural wisdom deals with the totality of life with reference to individual needs relating to physical and mental health, family structure, social situations, environment, and spiritual development.

Since most of you who will read or use the wisdom in this book may be influenced by modern medicine, therefore it is very important that I point out here the basic difference in the approach of these two systems. The modern medicine is based upon concept that the only cosmic reality is material and that can be approached with the senses. Further, the materials can be split into smaller fragments up to atoms and so on. Both, the cosmos and the human body work like a machine and the time is linear. Diseases, health and other events in life are dependent on chance factors. Contrary to that, the Āyurvedic approach is that the cosmos is a single dynamic, ever-changing whole where every function is for a definite purpose, where time is cyclic and it is a perfected system which works on cause, effect and its substratum. We human beings are a part of this big system in which our dynamic bodies and minds form a smaller system. We have discussed these concepts already in Section I of this book. Let me give you here, in brief, some concrete principles of Āyurveda and an outline of its practical aspects. For more details, you may consult my other books.[1]

For understanding the fundamental basis of Āyurveda, it is essential to understand the basic concept of *Sāṃkhya*, described in Section I. The story of Āyurveda begins from the five fundamental elements or *mahābhūtas* which form the material reality of the universe. These elements are ether, air, fire, water and earth and their equilibrium is essential for cosmic harmony and their imbalance and vitiation cause catastrophes in the world. The vitiation may be in the form of fast winds, fire accidents, too much heat, floods, earthquakes etc.

Since all what exists is made of five elements, it also includes human body. The same cosmic principles apply to it. But the body has soul in it, which is the cause of consciousness and makes it a vital organism. For the performance of vital functions, the five elements form three principal energies referred to as humours in English (*doṣa* in Sanskrit), and these are *vāta* from ether and air, *pitta* from fire and *kapha* from water and earth. These energies perform various mental and physical functions of the body and the nature of those functions depends upon the nature of the elements they originate from.

Vāta is responsible for entire body movements, blood circulation, respiration, excretion, speech, sensations, touch, hearing, feelings like fear, anxiety, grief, enthusiasm etc., natural urges, formation of foetus, sexual act and retention.

Pitta is responsible for vision, hunger, thirst, heat regulation, softness and lustre, cheerfulness, intellect and sexual vigour.

---

[1] My three books on Āyurveda have been published by Samuel Weiser, USA and the Indian editions of these books are as follows:

Āyurveda A Way of Life, 2001, Motilal Banarasidass, New Delhi,

Āyurveda for Life, Nutrition, Sexual Energy and Healing, 2001, Motilal Banarasidass, New Delhi.

Sixteen Minutes to a Better 9-to-5: Stress-free Work with Yoga and *Āyurveda*, 2000,

The fourth book is on women and their health (*The Kāmasūtra for Women*) published by Kodansha America and is recently published in India by Penguin-India, New Delhi.

Kapha constitutes all the solid structure of the body and is responsible for binding, firmness, heaviness, sexual potency, strength, forbearance and restraint.

Each person differs from another because of a slight difference in his or her fundamental constitution called *prakṛti*. This difference is due to the variation in the proportion of the three main energies. This variation is in terms of dominance of a particular humour or the combination of two humours. This is what makes us different from one another and unlike machines, as the system of modern medicine tends to make us. The *prakṛti* not only describes the variations in physiological features of individuals but also their personality types. Fundamental constitution of an individual is a very important theme of Āyurvedic wisdom and I have given some details of it in the box on next pages. For more details, consult my book, *Āyurveda: A Way of Life*.

For good health and long life, these three vital forces or humours should be in a state of equilibrium within their individual organisation as well as with respect to each other. However, if there is disturbance in one humour and it deviates from its quality, quantity or place or the three humours are not in proportion to each other, it leads to *vikṛti* or a state of vitiation, thus giving rise to various ailments. When the state of vitiation is left unattended for a long time, it may give rise to serious disorders.

Time, place, situation, nutrition, emotions etc. constantly influence humours or the vital forces and learning about the influence of these factors on your particular constitution, you can learn to maintain their equilibrium. These three vital forces are also related to our thought process and therefore it is foremost to keep equilibrium in the three qualities of the mind. The *rajas* quality of mind includes thinking, planning and taking decisions. The *tamas* quality is that which hinders motion and expansion of the mind (greed, anger, jealousy, laziness and so on). The *sattva* quality of mind includes equilibrium, goodness, truth, compassion, stillness and peace. The imbalance of *sattva*, *rajas* and *tamas* influences the equilibrium of the humours as well as causes mental ailments. Thus, for maintaining good health and longevity, a six-dimensional equilibrium is essential as these three dimensions at two levels influence each other. The imbalance of these three qualities of mind also influences the equilibrium of humours and vice versa.

PRAKṚTI OR THE INDIVIDUAL CONSTITUTION

A mother observes differences in the personality traits of her two babies from the beginning and the siblings differ in their likes and dislikes of food products, their reaction to weather and climate, the effect of drugs, the fundamental way of reacting to situations and other personality traits. According to Āyurveda, each one of us has an individual constitution from the birth. It is the basis of our physiological and psychological reactions. For maintaining good health and equilibrium, it is essential to take the individual constitution into consideration.

Prakṛti of an individual is due to the dominance of one or more humours and attributes the individual the characteristics of that particular humour in slightly more predominance than the others. For example, the *pitta prakṛti* individuals will be more sensitive to heat, sweat more and eat and drink more. The *vāta prakṛti* ones are more agile and swift in their movements. The *kapha prakṛti* persons are slow and stable in their movements and are more tolerant than the previous two. In the mixed *prakṛti*, the person may experience different attributes at different times.

Seven type of *prakṛti*

vāta	*vāta-pitta*	*vāta-kapha*
pitta	*pitta-kapha*	
kapha	*Samadoṣā* (all humours in equal proportions)	

The difference in the proportions of the humours is one factor of variation. Their degree is another factor. For example, one may be slightly *vāta* dominating or in various upward grades. The proportion of the two humours may vary in the mixed *prakṛti*. The fundamental presence of the grade of these three energies is another varying factor. For example, there are some individuals with plenty of energy, tremendous stamina and vitality, very good immune system and a brilliant mind. These persons have basically all the three energies or humours in high grade. Then comes the domination of one or more and forms their *prakṛti*.

If we imagine the fundamental presence of the three energies on a scale of 10 and then multiply them with seven types of *prakṛti*, we get a large number of human types. Further on, in each case, the degree of dominance is also considered and in mixed *prakṛti*, the proportion of the two humours is also taken into consideration, we will end up with numerous sorts of *prakṛti*.

Importance of *prakṛti*

Since all in this cosmos is made of five elements including our body and everything is interconnected and interdependent, the outer factors influence us constantly. To maintain the equilibrium of five elements in the body, which are present in the form of three humours, it is essential that an individual knows his or her constitution. If a person with predominant fire element (*pitta prakṛti*) does actions or consumes foods with the dominance of the same element, he or she may end up in getting this energy vitiated and may fall ill. Therefore, to know one's *prakṛti* is essentail for using the Āyurvedic wisdom. For nutrition, weather, geographical location as well as remedies, *prakṛti* or the fundamental constitution is taken into consideration.

With external factors like nutrition, geographical location and lifestyle, one can alter the vitiation and proportion of the humours but the basic individual constitution does not alter. However, in pathological situations such as an illness or accidental injuries, one may temporarily acquire different traits than one's *prakṛti,* but getting cured, the usual features by which one is charctrerised, come back. For example, if you are having *vāta prakṛti* and due to some sickness, you sleep a lot, become slow in your movements and so on, after getting cured, you will automatically acquire your ususal swiftness.

The basic human nature does not change, the variations may occur due to life situations. Imagine someone *pitta* dominating who is impatient and gets angry very quickly, and has also a *pitta* dominating partner. This couple may have fights, confrontations and disputes. Being similar, both these individuals will tend to enhance and aggravate each other's anger. Later in life, imagine one of them living with a *kapha* predominant person with patience and tolerance. Gradually, this *pitta* dominant person will lessen his anger. The other person's patience gives time to think and reflect and not to react.

Besides being important for health and healing, the knowledge of the *prakṛti* of individuals can lead us to better understaning of each other in family life, at work place and in other aspects of social interaction.

In Tables 7, 8 and 9, I have given some details about the three humours. There are characteristics of domination of a humour, the factors, which vitiate them, symptoms of vitiation and the remedies for that. These tables are taken from my book *Āyurveda: A Way of Life.*

The six-dimensional equilibrium

Our state of mind influences our principal energies, which are responsible for physical and mental functions of the body. For example, if we are worried or are over-worked or have a hectic mental state, *vāta* gets vitiated and some symptoms of its vitiation appear (Table 7). Too much anger influences *pitta* and one can suffer from *pitta* related disorders like stomach ailments (Table 8). Depression gives rise to *kapha* related disorders leading to obesity, nausea, excessive salivation and so on (Table 9).

When a humour vitiates and there are related disorders, they in turn influence the mental state of an individual. If constipation or partial evacuation persists, it can give rise to sleep disorders or hectic mental state or nervous behaviour. Stomach problems, which are due to *pitta* disturbances, may enhance anger and irritation.

Thus, it is important to understand that in Āyurveda, for keeping basic equilibrium of the body, the efforts at six-dimensional level are required. One cannot think of doing everything relating to the three humours and expect to be in perfect health. Equally important is to maintain a mental level of equilibrium with a state of happiness and satisfaction. We come to this theme once again in the last section of the book.

Prakṛti and *vikṛti*

For the understanding of the Āyurvedic principles, this is a very important concept to comprehend. *Prakṛti* means nature and in Āyurveda, as described above, it refers to a person's individual nature, that is the individual constitution in terms of physiological and psychological personality of an individual. According to natural cosmic principles, the nature of the body is to be healthy. The individual variations account for the diversity in nature of different persons. The basic equilibrium of the three humours should be maintained for health and harmony. This equilibrium is constantly influenced by external factors like weather, climate, place, time

Table 7. The origin, functions and characteristics of *Vāta.*

Vāta is light, subtle, mobile, dry, cold, rough, and all-pervasive, like the basic elements (Air and Ether) from which it is derived.

↓

Vāta is responsible for body movement and mind activity, blood circulation, respiration, excretion, speech, sensation, touch, hearing, feelings (like fear, anxiety, grief, enthusiasm, etc.), natural urges, formation of the fetus, sexual act, and retention.

Vāta-dominating people

- Agile;
- Quick and unrestricted in their movements;
- Swift in action;
- Quick in fear, and other emotions;
- Gets easily irritated;
- Intolerant to cold and shivers easily;
- Coarse hairs and nails;
- Prominent blood vessels.

Factors which increase *Vāta*

- Fasting;
- Excessive physical exercise;
- Exposure to cold;
- Laziness;
- Staying awake late at night;
- Rainy season;
- Old age;
- Evening and last part of the night;
- Eating over-ripened, dry food which is kept a long time after cooking;
- Injury;
- Blood loss;
- Excessive sexual intercourse;
- Anxiety;
- Uneven posture;
- Suppression of natural urges;
- Guilt.

Signs of vitiated *Vāta*

- General stiffness and pain in the body;
- Bad taste and dryness in the mouth;
- Lack of appetite;
- Stomach ache;
- Dry skin;
- Fatigue;
- Dark-coloured stool;
- Insomnia;
- Pain in temporal region;
- Giddiness;
- Tremors;
- Yawning;
- Hiccups;
- Malaise;
- Delirium;
- Dull complexion;
- Withdrawn and timid behaviour.

Treatment of vitiated *Vāta*

- Sweet, sour and hot therapeutic measures;
- Enema;
- *Vāta*-decreasing diet;
- Massage;
- Anointing;
- Appropriate rest, relaxation and sleep;
- Peaceful atmosphere;
- Cheerful mental state.

Table 8. The origin, functions and characteristics of *Pitta.*

Pitta is hot like the basic element (fire) from which it is derived. Its characteristics are sharp, sour, pungent and it has a fleshy smell.

↓

Pitta is responsible for vision, digestion, hunger and thirst, heat regulation, softness and luster, cheerfulness, intellect and sexual vigour.

Pitta-dominating people

- Intolerant to heat;
- Have usually hot faces;
- Delicate organs;
- Tendency to have moles, freckles, pimples (acne);
- Lustrous complexion;
- Excessive hunger and thirst;
- Early appearance of wrinkles;
- Falling and graying hairs;
- Body smell;
- Intolerance and lack of endurance.

Factors which increase *Pitta*

- Sharp, alkaline, salty foods;
- Any food or drink that creates burning sensations;
- Sunbathing;
- Noon time;
- Midnight;
- Autumn;
- Process of digestion;
- Youth;
- Anger.

Signs of vitiated *Pitta*

- Excessive perspiration;
- Smell in the body;
- Abnormal hunger and thirst;
- Inflammation;
- Tearing and thickening of skin;
- Rash;
- Acne;
- Herpes;
- Excessive heat in the body;
- Burning sensation;
- Loss of contentment
- Dissatisfaction;
- Anger.

Treatment of vitiated *Pitta*

- Sweet, bitter, astringent, and cold measures;
- Unction and purgation;
- Fasting;
- Cold baths and massage;
- Special *Pitta*-decreasing diets;
- Consolation.

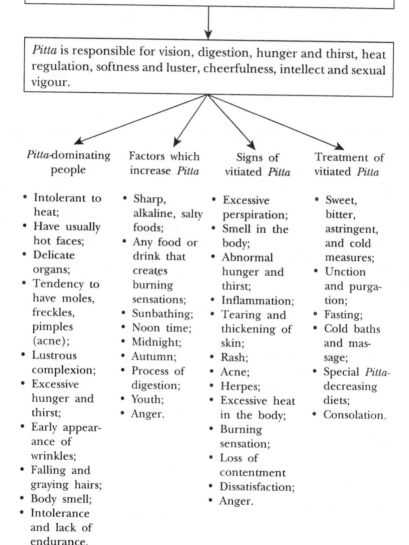

Table 9. The origin, functions and characteristics of *Kapha*.

Kapha is derived from the basic elements (Earth and Water) and like these elements it is soft, solid, dull, sweet, heavy, cold, slimy, unctuous and immobile.

Kapha constitutes the solid structure of the body and is responsible for unctuousness, binding, firmness, heaviness, sexual potency, strength, forbearance, restraint and the absence of greed.

Kapha-dominating people

- Dull in activities, diet, and speech;
- Delayed initiation;
- Disorderly;
- Stable movements;
- Well-united and strong ligaments;
- Little hunger, thirst, or perspiration;
- Clear eyes, face, and complexion

Factors which increase *Kapha*

- Salty, alkaline foods;
- Oily, fatty, heavy to digest nutrients;
- Sedentary life style;
- Lack of exercise;
- Daydreaming;
- Childhood;
- Spring season;
- Morning time;
- First part of the night.

Signs of vitiated *Kapha*

- Drowsiness;
- Excessive sleep;
- Sweet taste in the mouth;
- Excessive salivation;
- Heaviness in the body;
- Cold sensation;
- Nausea;
- Itchy feelings in the throat;
- Whiteness in urine, eyes, and faeces;
- Deformed body organs;
- Weariness;
- Lassitude;
- Inertness and depression.

Treatment of vitiated *Kapha*

- Pungent, bitter, astringent, sharp, hot and rough measures;
- Wet heat;
- Vomiting
- Exercise;
- Keeping awake;
- *Kapha*-decreasing diet.

(age, time of the day and time of the year), nutrition, social interaction, work and so on. I have illustrated some of these factors in Tables 10, and Figure 13, which are cited from my previously published book, *Āyurveda for Life.* It is also influenced by internal factors like our thoughts and reactions, body postures and living style. A person should make an effort to live according to time and place and follow other principles to be in harmony with cosmic as well as internal influences to maintain the fundamental nature of the body and mind. Due to weather, emotions, nutrition and other allied factors, we may divert from the state of *prakṛti* (health) to *vikṛti* (state of non-health). Āyurveda teaches us to take various steps to get out of the state of *vikṛti* and to regain the state of *prakṛti.* With knowledge and through personal effort, we can bring ourselves to the state of *prakṛti* again. However, if the

Table 10. The humours and the environment

HUMOURS IN RELATION TO SEASONS	
Season	**Dominating Humours**
Rainy	*Vāta*
Warm and Dry (Summer and Autumn)	*Pitta*
Cold (Winter)	*Kapha*
HUMOURS IN RELATION TO AGE	
Age	**Dominating Humours**
Childhood	*Kapha*
Youth	*Pitta*
Old Age	*Vāta*
HUMOURS IN RELATION TO PLACE	
Place	**Dominating Humours**
Forest	*Vāta*
Desert	*Vāta-Pitta*
Mountains	*Vāta-Kapha*
Coastal Areas	*Kapha-Pitta*
Midlands	None

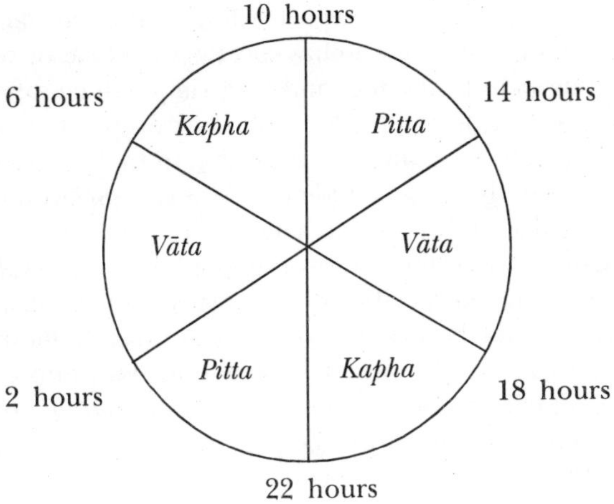

Figure 13. Various parts of the day in relation to humours

state of non-health is allowed to persist, it gradually creates more imbalance in the body and over a period of time, there are one or more disorders. Thus, for maintaining good health and avoiding ailments, one should be able to recognise the state of *vikṛti* and do all to re-establish the harmony and to get to the state of *prakṛti*.

According to Āyurveda, one should make best of one's efforts to prevent ailments and disorders. Despite all efforts, if there are health problems, they should be treated in a holistic manner with three-dimensional therapy of Āyurveda and after the ailment is cured, the balance should be re-established by appropriate medication. After treatment, the patient should be given *rasāyanas* to rebuild the immunity and vitality of the body.

Āyurvedic nutrition

Nutrition plays an extremely important role in healing as well as making people sick. We observe that millions of people around the world are over-fed and obese and suffer from various ailments due to malnutrition in the direction of excessive nutrition. Contrary to this, in the Southern Hemisphere of the globe, there are drought, hunger, wars and famine and many people suffer from malnutrition in the sense of under-nutrition. The nutrients can be healing or poisonous for us according to the time and need. For example for someone who has sweat a lot in heat or otherwise and is getting pain in the legs and feet, simply some salted water with lemon and sugar is a healer. The same preparation will have a negative effect on someone suffering from hypertension or diabetes. Cold milk is good for persons with *pitta prakṛti* and during summer months. On the other hand, milk taken by a person of *kapha prakṛti* during winter nights is enough to cause *kapha vikṛti.*

There are detailed specifications in Āyurveda for nutrients and their effect on our bodies in reference to three humours. With knowledge of Āyurvedic wisdom about nutrition, one can treat oneself to get back the lost balance and regain the state of *prakṛti.* There are nutrients, which can be preventive for certain ailments and the others which have a curative effect.

Principles of Āyurvedic nutrition

The basic equilibrium of nutrition and the humours

Body as well as nutrients are made of five elements. In the body, the five elements constitute three principal energies or humours that perform all physical and mental functions of the body. In the nutrients, there are six principal *rasa* or tastes which are derived from two elements each. Through nutrients, we supply the body with elements, which in turn form the three principal energies (*vāta, pitta* and *kapha*). We need the supply of these three energies constantly in our bodies as they are also consumed for performing various functions.

For good health and harmony, we require maintaining the balance of the three humours or energies. This balance should be maintained by consuming the six *rasas* in appropriate proportions so that we have a balanced supply of the five fundamental elements in our bodies, which in turn will create the equilibrium of humours. Each *rasa* reacts on our bodies according to the elements it is made of. For example, sweet is from water and earth and it brings *kapha* to the body. Sour is from fire and water and it brings both *pitta* and *kapha.* The five elements balance each other according to their characteristics. For example, sweet that contains water and earth also appeases the excessive fire or excessive *vāta* which is dry in nature.

The idea of balanced nutrition is illustrated in Figure 14. This figure is from my book *Sixteen Minutes to a Better* 9-to-5.

Nutrition according to prakṛti, time and space

The above description of the Āyurvedic nutrition tells us about the basic principle. There are other external and internal factors, which have to be taken into consideration. The major internal factor is the individual constitution or *prakṛti.* The individuals with different constitutions need to lay emphasis on different kinds of foods. In the living tradition of Āyurveda, this aspect is dealt with in a very simple manner. The nutrients are cold, hot or in equilibrium as for their Āyurvedic nature is concerned. Combinations of cold and hot lead to balance. The nutrients, which are in equilibrium are easy to digest and are health promoting. Nutrients which are extremely cold and extremely hot in their Āyurvedic properties should not be consumed without creating an equilibrium in them with the help of specific spices of consuming them with other foods which bring equilibrium by their opposite Āyurvedic properties. Āyurveda provides us a list of antagonist nutrients that should be strictly avoided.

Another category of internal factors may originate from the state of mind. Emotions like worry, fear, excitement etc. may cause an imbalance of *vāta,* anger may cause imbalance of *pitta* and depression may give rise to an imbalance of *kapha.* Thus, one should have nutrition according to the circumstances in order to maintain equilibrium. If someone is already a little depressed, eats sweet, cold, heavy and oily diet, that will enhance the problems. Eating in a state of anger gives rise to *pitta* related disorders. Cool and light diet after the suppression of anger should be taken. The emotional state of mind, which leads to *vāta* imbalance, should be appeased with sweet, warm and unctuous diet.

Nutrition should co-ordinate with time of the day, time of the year, one's age and the geographical location. These are the external factors that influence us and the variations due to these are already shown in Table 10 and in Figure 13.

For more details of nutriton, you may consult my book, *Āyurveda for Life: Nutrition, Sexual Energy and Healing.* My forthcoming book, *Āyurvedic Food Culture and Recipes* (Samuel Weiser USA and Penguin-India) provides more details of the Āyurvedic nutrition in all its practical aspects.

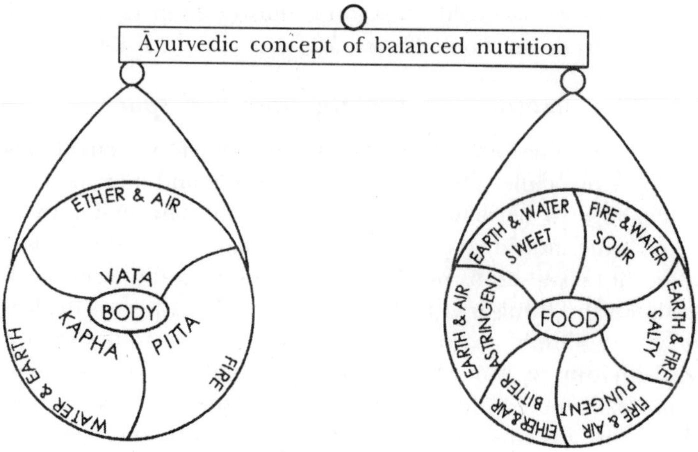

Figure 14. Āyurvedic concept of balanced nutrition

External purification and internal purification (*Pañcakarma*) practices of Āyurveda

In Āyurveda, both internal and external purification practices are very important for maintaining good health, beauty, vigour and longevity. These practices not only purify the organisms, but they are also meant to rejuvenate and insure proper functions of the body. I have summed up below the principal purification practices suggested in Āyurveda and have also given some suggestions in the context of our modern life-style.

External purification

1. **General purification of the morning:** Drink about half litre of warm water upon getting up in the morning and some yogic exercises or a walk should follow this.
2. **Cleaning mouth, teeth and tongue:** While brushing your teeth, clean your tongue properly with a soft brush or a tongue cleaner. Dirty tongue gives rise to a foul smell. Each time you eat something, rinse your mouth with water and if it is not possible immediately, eat a cardamom or clove to purify your mouth cavity. It is suggested to eat 4-5 cardamoms a day for perfuming the mouth and strengthening the teeth.

3. **Cleaning the nasal passage:** Clear the nasal passage for the free flow of vital air (*prāṇa* energy), blow always your nose strongly after your shower. Dip two of your fingers in mustard oil, insert them into your nasal passage and inhale. This exercise will make you sneeze and clear your nasal passage.
4. **Ears:** The sticky secretion of the ears should be cleaned from time to time. The outer ear should be thoroughly cleaned while taking shower and should be given an oil massage.
5. **Eyes:** Upon getting up in the morning, the eyes should be splashed with cold water. It is recommended to use mild eye-drops for cleaning the eyes time to time. Use of honey in the eyes before going to bed is highly recommended. The honey should be pure and of good quality.
6. **Skin:** Soaps and shampoos dry the skin and therefore you should clean your body with full cream milk from time to time. Rub the body with raw milk and wash it away with water. When using soaps, mix them with some oil or oil your body before or after using the soap.
7. **Head and hair:** The scalp gets very dry with the constant use of shampoos. It is recommended to have a coconut or sesames or olive oil massage on your head and leave it for several hours before shampooing your hair. After washing, rinse the hair with liquorice decoction or a mixture of lemon juice and honey in the ratio of 1:2.
8. **Vagina:** Wash the vagina with vaginal douche or enema apparatus using some bitter decoction like neem or bitter gourd (*karelā*).

Internal purifications or Pañcakarma

The classical *pañcakarma* includes:

1. Emesis (vomiting)
2. Purgation
3. Non-unctuous enema
4. Unctuous enemas
5. *Nasya* or the purification of the head region

Before doing the *pañcakarma* practices, some preparatory practices are required. These are different kinds of oil massages, dry and wet fomentation and intake of fat. These are essential for extracting the toxins from the body with ease through the above-described practices. After each of the cleansing practices, a specific diet and care is also essential.

It is recommended that these practices should be performed twice a year after two major seasons, after the summer and winter. These help to throw away the imbalances and keep one healthy and vigorous. For curative purposes, the major imbalances in the body that cause nagging ailments can be uprooted through the internal purifications. If these disorders are cured with medications, their root may remain inside the body and they may recur. With the internal purification practices, they are completely eradicated. For handling disorders, the *pañcakarma* practices should be done under the supervision of a competent physician or should be learnt and understood from a *vaidya.*

Relationship of the three humours to *pañcakarma*

Enemas are the principal cure for *vāta* vitiation and the disorders caused by that. The major treatment for *pitta* vitiation and its allied disorders is purgation. The main treatment for an imbalance of *kapha* and the resulting ailments is done with emesis. *Nasya* or the purification of the head region cures the ailments of head region relating to any of the three humours.

A regular half-yearly purification throws out the imbalance of any of these humours from the body and saves one from the disorders caused due to the internal imbalance in the body. It also rejuvenates the body organs and gives rise to beauty and vigour. However, the purification practices should be done in an appropriate and systematic manner. If they are done without proper precautions and pre-treatments like massage, fomentation etc., they can be harmful for you. Besides, there are other precautions to be taken which are related to age, constitution and other specific conditions of the body. For more practical details, you may consult my books *Āyurveda for Life* and *Sixteen Minutes to a Better* 9-to-5.

From *pañcakarma* to *saptakarma*

Keeping in view our modern times with *prāṇa vikṛti* due to air pollution and noise pollution, intake of various chemical sprays through our food and consumption of chemical drugs by a large majority of population, I have added two more purification practices to the classical five practices. These are blood purification and diuresis (purification of the kidneys, bladder etc.). Blood purification or blood detoxification is done with a combination of certain plant drugs taken twice a year for 15 days. This practice will save us from the negative effects of the pollutants we consume knowingly or unknowingly and from some of their allergic reactions.

Diuresis is done by the intake of a plant product which is diuretic in nature, accompanied by drinking lot of liquid to flush out any deposits of dirt inside kidneys or bladder.

Purification of the uterus and breasts

According to Āyurveda, women should do purification of the parts related to their womanhood. This is done with specific plants many of which are a part of everyday life in Indian households. This purification should be particularly recommended before pregnancy, after childbirth and during menopausal years. For details of this theme, you may consult my book, *The Kāmasūtra for Women.*

Disease and therapy in Āyurveda

It is important to understand the fundamentals of disease and therapy in Āyurveda to comprehend the application of its principles. Both disease and therapy are looked upon from a very different point of view as most of you are used to from modern medicine (allopathy). Body is not treated as a machine and a disease does not come by chance. They are the results of our present or previous *karma* or due to a lack of emotional equilibrium. A disease or a disorder is built gradually in the body and does not come suddenly, although it may appear like that sometimes.

Three types of diseases

There are three types of diseases: innate, exogenous and psychic (Table 11). Innate diseases are those that arise due to imbalance of three humours, like diabetes, several types of aches and pains, different digestive disorders etc. These are caused by a long-term imbalance of the body's three principal energies due to an erroneous way of living. The second category of disorders is exogenous and are due to external factors like pollutants, toxins,

Table 11. Three categories of diseases according to Āyurveda.

THREE TYPES OF DISEASE		
Innate	**Exogenous**	**Psychic**
Innate diseases are those that arise due to imbalance in three humours–*Vāta, Pitta, Kapha.*	Exogenous diseases are those that arise due to external factors, such as poisons, polluted air, parasites, bacteria, viruses, etc.	Psychic diseases are those caused by unfulfillment of desires or facing the undesired.

bacteria, virus or other parasites or due to accidents. The third category of disorders is psychic and they are caused by the non-fulfilment of desires and facing the undesired.

These three types of disorders are interrelated. The imbalance of the three energies diminishes one's *ojas* (immunity and vitality) and makes one vulnerable to external disorders. Innate and exogenous disorders cause weakness and make one mentally feeble. The mental weakness makes one less tolerant and irritable and gives rise to a state of dissatisfaction leading to more complicated health problems. The lack of control over one's mind has a similar effect.

The important messages from Āyurveda for the prevention of the ailments are the following:

1. According to the Āyurvedic principles, one should do every effort to create a balance of the three humours and the three qualities of the mind (see above: the six dimensional equilibrium).
2. One should take rejuvenating products, the *rasāyanas,* in order to enhance one's immunity and vitality so that one is able to prevent the exogenous disorders.
3. One should do the half-yearly purification practices and follow other life-style recommendations of Āyurveda for the same purpose.

4. One should learn to keep control on one's mental activities through yogic practices and learn to acquire a state of satisfaction or *santoṣa* so that one is able to avoid the psychic disorders.

Three-dimensional therapy of Āyurveda

Āyurveda recommends three-dimensional therapy in case of an ailment. These three kinds of therapies are rational, psychological and spiritual and they should be applied simultaneously. We can also apply these principles to maintain the state of health, to cure our minor ailments and to prevent disease. The three-dimensional therapy is illustrated in Table 12.

Natural urges and their relation to health

According to Āyurveda, the natural human urges are divided into two categories, suppressible and non-suppressible. The non-suppressible urges are natural biological needs and if they are suppressed, the body suffers from temporary disorders, which should be cured with appropriate measures. The suppressible urges belong to our mind and by developing mental discipline, they should be suppressed. If they are not suppressed, they give rise to a dissatisfied mental state and ultimately cause ill health and physical and mental disorders. Table 13 illustrates this theme. This is a brief description of the principles of Āyurveda. These pages are not meant to be a guide for you for an Āyurvedic way of life and nor this is for a complete comprehension of the subject. That is the reason why I have referred to my various books as reference material for further reading. As far as *pañcakarma* is concerned, many volumes have been written on this subject. For treating serious disorders and diseases through *pañcakarma*, a very experienced and specialised physician is required. For normal purification methods, you may learn to perform these practices yourself. In any case, if you wish to adopt Āyurvedic way of life on your own, it is essential to get more knowledge through books and teachers.

Table 12. The three-dimensional therapy of Āyurveda

Rational therapy

Rational therapy involves right kind of diet and drugs, appropriate rest, outer and inner cleaning practices, massage, anointing, appropriate physical exercise, congenial atmosphere for recovery, climate change etc.

Psychological therapy

Pschological therapy comprises of using mental effort and energy to participate in the process of recovery. Thought process is directed towards searching the causes of the ailment and factors that enhance it. The mind's effort and will power is used to eradicate them. In case the patient is weak to use his/her mental energy, mental support and courage should be provided by the physician or some other person who is trustworthy for the patient. For maintaining the state of health we can also direct our mental energy in this direction.

Spiritual therapy

Spiritual therapy consists of recitation of mantras, wearing roots and gems, auspicious acts, offerings, oblations, following religious precepts, atonement, fasting, invoking blessings, rendering oneself to gods, offerings, donations, pilgrimage and other similar acts. Roots, seeds and gems etc. are used for spiritual therapy because they are supposed to have specific cosmic energy and to carry them on human body influences the body's subtle energy. Such things are brought from holy places and holy persons after invoking their blessings. Through prayers, pilgrimage and worship, human consciousness recognises the cosmic power beyond the material reality and is able to establish a connection with the limitless, timeless and endless energy.

Table 13. Non-suppressible and suppressible natural urges

NATURAL URGES

- Non-suppressible
  - Urge of urine feces, semen, flatus, vomiting, sneezing, eructation, yawning, hunger, thirst, tears, sleep and breathing fast after exertion.
- Suppressible
  - Urge of evil ventures relating to thought, speech and action; urge of greed, grief, fear, anger, vanity, envy, excessive attachment.

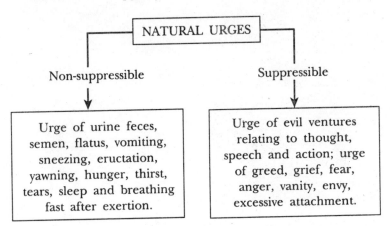

SECTION IV

Integration of Yoga and Āyurveda

Holistic living

When my first book on Āyurveda appeared in 1992, many people were quite surprised to find the importance of yogic practices in *Āyurvedic way of life.* The modern reductionist approach to health care practices as well as the fragmented way of living makes people extend this similar outlook on a holistic system. In a holistic way of living, it is not possible that different disciplines are disintegrated. If it is that, the system is no more holistic. Everything in the cosmos is interrelated, interconnected and interdependent. Our being is a part of this whole system. The disciplines we create have to be a part of the cosmic rhythm of which our being (body, mind and soul) is a part. I will explain this statement in the context of the Indian tradition of which Āyurveda is a part. Āyurveda is created for good health, longevity and curing ailments. Its principles are based upon cosmic principles of harmony and balance of the five fundamental elements. It suggests that for healthy living, one should be in harmony with space and time. Designing cities and houses is termed as *vāstu* (architecture). To be in harmony with space and time, the human habitations should also be designed by applying the same cosmic principles. How can human beings be in tune with the cosmic energy if the houses they live in are not built according to the same principles?

Through our food, we constantly provide five elements to our body, which in turn constitute three vital forces (the humours) for performing all the physical and mental functions of the body. Our food gets these five elements (ether, air, fire, water, and earth) directly from the cosmic energy. When with advanced (?) food technology, we grow our food with artificial chemical fertilizers and other such means, naturally, that food will be inappropriate to provide us the required vitality, leading to various deformities and disorders in the body. Thus, the discipline of agriculture also has to be developed keeping in view the fundamental cosmic principles.

Since antiquity, it is well known that our way of living, thinking and behaviour directly affects our health and with a peaceful and relaxed state of mind, the healing process is accelerated. The Greeks built the great healing resorts with theatre, music and other arts. The arts directly affect the human mind and the great Indian theory of art appreciation is derived from the *rasa* theory of Āyurveda. Our body is made of five fundamental elements and so are the *rasa* in our food. If we do not include all the *rasa* in our food, we create an imbalance of the five elements in our body, thus leading to humoral imbalance and causing ailments. Similarly, if we continue to entertain ourselves with works of arts, which only evoke certain set of emotions in us, we can create a mental imbalance. For example, if we watch continuously films and theatres related to horror and crime or listen to rapid and hectic music, we can make ourselves sick due to *vāta* and *rajas* imbalance.

Sāṃkhya, yoga and Āyurveda

Patañjali's yoga is a practical application of *Sāṃkhya.* Patañjali provides us techniques to reach the ultimate goal of achieving eternity unfolded by *Sāṃkhya.* I have said earlier that both yoga and Āyurveda have their fundamental basis in *Sāṃkhya.* In Āyurvedic literature, the concepts of *Sāṃkhya* are mentioned and this wisdom is interpreted in reference to the human body.

> **"Again from division of constituents, the *Puruṣa* is known as possessing twenty-four entities such as mind, ten sense organs and organs of action, five fundamental elements and *Prakṛti* along with intellect, individuating principle and five sense objects."[1]**

The body has been analysed in terms of *Sāṃkhya* as follows:

> **"The five fundamental elements along with intellect, individuating principle and *prakṛti* (eight constituents) make the original source of creatures (*bhūtaprakṛti*). Mind, five sense objects, five sense organs, five organs of action (sixteen constituents) are the *vikāras* or the products. This aggregate of the twenty-four elements is known as *kṣetra* (field) or the body. The soul or the unmanifest is known as the knower of this body by the sages."[2]**

1 *Caraka Saṃhitā, Śarīrasthānam,* I, 17
2 *Ibid,* I, 63-67

In Āyurveda it is said that **"There is no beginning of the self (soul) and there is continuity of the created body; it is impossible to say which is earlier."**[3] Continuity of the body is in the form of the cycle of birth and death. Patañjali has stated in Sūtra 13 of Part II that the birth, rank etc. in the next life are decided according to the results of the previous *karma* and that an individual acquires a body with the qualities resulting from those. That is how the ancient sages have seen the continuity of the body.

As in yoga, conceit, fear, anger etc. are hindrance in the way of achieving the goal of yoga, similarly these are obstacles for achieving good health. According to Caraka:

> **"Conceit, fear, anger, greed, ignorance, narcosis and confusion, troublesome actions taken under spell and other actions arisen from *rajas* and *tamas* are due to intellectual error and are the cause of diseases."**[4]

The first five parts of Patañjali's eight-fold yoga are forebearance, self-discipline, yogic postures (*yogāsana*), breathing practices (*prāṇāyāma*) and restraint (see Table 5 for the eight yogic practices). These five practices are preparatory to the last three practices, which are attention, contemplation and meditation. The first five practices belong to our external world of which our body is a part whereas the last three belong to our inner being. The first five practices of yoga are in a way preparatory to the rest three to achieve the goal of yoga, i.e. *kaivalya.* The first five practices are related to the body and the other aspects of our being in relation to our social surroundings. During our ephemeral existence on this planet; the body is the cause of involvement in the world. On the other hand, the path to freedom is only possible through the body. Therefore, body or our physical being is of prime importance in yoga. Āyurveda is the science of life and obviously deals with all aspects of life and reveals the wisdom for having an optimum, disease-free, happy and harmonious existence. Thus, yoga and Āyurveda come together for the well-being of the body. However, in yoga, the well-being of the body is with a specific aim in mind whereas in Āyurveda, the aim depends upon the individual's discretion–it may be for enjoying the worldly pleasures or for some other purpose.

---

3 *Caraka Saṃhitā, Śarīrasthānam,* I, 82

4 *Ibid,* I, 109

Table 14. Caraka's interpretation of human existence according to the *Sāṃkhya* principles.

HUMAN EXISTENCE

Bhūtaprakṛti	***Vikāras***
(The original source of creatures) is constituted of eight elements	(The products of the *bhūtaprakṛti*) are constituted of sixteen elements
↓	↓
Prakṛti	Mind
Intellect	Five sense objects: Sound, Touch, Appearance, Flavour, Odour
Individuating principle	Five sense organs: Hearing, Feeling, Seeing, Tasting, Smelling
Five fundamental elements: Ether, Air, Fire, Water, Earth	Five organs of action: Express, Grasp, Move, Excrete, Procreate

The aggregate of these twenty-four elements constitutes the physical being known as *kṣetra* or field. The twenty-fifth element is soul which is the cause of consciousness or puts life in the body and is known as 'the knower of the field'.

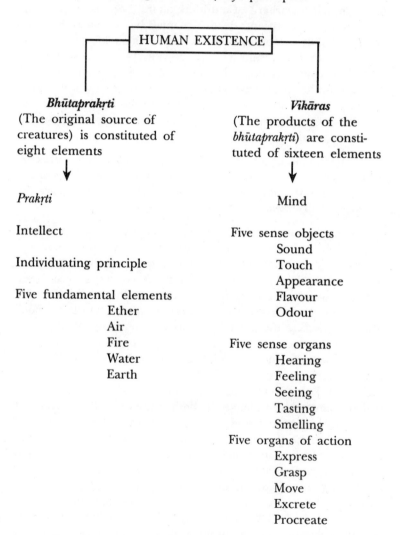

Another aspect where yoga and Āyurveda have oneness (though their aims are different) is the effect of *karma.* The aim of yoga is to get rid of the previous *karma* and their effect in the form of *saṃskāra* in order to attain freedom from the cycle of birth and death. All this is achieved with tremendous personal effort. The purpose of Āyurveda is to get rid of the bad effect of the previous *karma,* which comes to us in the form of disease (termed as *daiva* in Āyurveda). In this case also, the emphasis is laid on the personal effort that is made at physical, mental and spiritual levels (termed as *puruṣakāra* in Āyurveda). Thus, the basic rationale of Āyurvedic cure is the same as that of yoga. If with yogic practices or *sādhanā,* the remains of previous *karma* (*saṃskāra*) can be dissolved, then with similar practices it must also be possible to nullify the effect of the previous *karma* which comes to us in the form of ailment or disease. The use of will power, persistence to achieve the aim, appropriate and regular medication which helps to get rid of the ailment is also a kind of *sādhanā,* though with a different aim. For maintaining good health, one has to keep equilibrium between *daiva* and *puruṣakāra.* That means that as far as health is concerned, our present *karma* have to be according to the need of our state of health which we brought with us from previous *karma.* For example, if someone has weak health from childhood and tends to get ill frequently, this person has to make specific efforts to take *rasāyanas* to enhance the *ojas* (immunity and vitality) and take precautions and medications to prevent and heal ailments. On the other hand, if some-one is blessed with extremely good health, stamina and intellect due to his/her previous *karma,* this person has relatively lesser effort to make. Nevertheless everything should be done to maintain that vigour until the old age, if the health is taken for granted and nothing is done, the stock of previous *karma* may deplete. Personal effort or *puruṣakāra* is very important for every-one and more so for those who have already health problems. We are all born with different conditions at the time of birth in the context of health, wealth, family status etc. due to our previous *karma.* Let us take two extreme examples in the context of health. Some of us may be born with palace and the other with ruins. With negligence, one can bring the palace (extremely good health) to ruin and with tremendous personal efforts, one can make at least a small house out of a ruin.

There are two principal differences between Patañjali's yoga and Āyurveda. Yoga has a deterministic view on the age of an individual (*Yogasūtra*, Section II, Sūtra 13) whereas Āyurveda has no basis to exist if age, disease etc. are predestined. According to Caraka:

> **"If there be a determined life span, there would not be any necessity to apply mantras, medicines, gems, auspicious rites, offering, gifts, observance of rules, expiation, fasting etc... with a desire for longevity. Nor there would be any need to avoid excited and fierce cows, elephants, horses, camels, asses, buffaloes and terrific winds etc. Likewise, one will not abstain from waterfalls, mountains, uneven and difficult places, strong water currents or from careless, excited, fierce and insane persons, from those inflicted with confusion and greed, from enemies, from furious fire, from various poisonous reptiles and snakes etc."**[5]

Thus, we see very strong opinion of Caraka against the deterministic view of the life span and his rationale for abandoning this view. Indeed, the bases of health care practices are lost if we believe that the age and the ailments are predetermined. I will explain more on *karma* and Āyurveda a little later in this Section.

The second difference between yoga and Āyurveda is about *ahiṃsa* or not killing and paining. First of the eight yogic practices (*yama*) has one part which forbids killing and causing pain to others directly or indirectly (*Yogasūtra*, Part II, Sūtra 34). Āyurveda does not take a moral stand on this issue but has a neutral opinion about meat eating which obviously involves paining and killing. There is a detailed description of numerous edibles from the animal kingdom and their effect on the three humours[6]. There are details of the seafood, frogs, various kinds of eggs, meats from all sorts of animals including wild animals. There are also details of the Āyurvedic nature of different parts of the animals. We must understand that Āyurveda is science of life and it takes a neutral point of view; it gives us description of all possible edible substances around us. It does not tell us about a moral path; it is

---

5 *Caraka Saṃhitā, Vimānasthānam*, III, 36.

6 For details of this theme, refer to my book, *Āyurveda for Life: Nutrition, Sexual Energy and Healing*.

left to an individual's sense of discretion. The second aspect is that there are parts of our globe which do not have enough edible substances of plant origin to cater to the need of local population throughout the year and it becomes necessary to eat meat products in such regions. Tibet is a good example in this context. Despite being Buddhist (Buddhism propagates *ahiṃsā* very strongly), the Tibetans have to eat meat as in the high Himalayan regions there is not much vegetation.

Karma and Āyurveda

I have described above that according to both yoga and Āyurveda, we have to deal with the results of our past *karma*. First of all, let me make clear that the past *karma* are not necessarily from the past life or lives. They can be from the recent past. In fact, when we talk of past life or lives, we merely see time in a bigger scale. To understand the effect of *karma* and the interaction of past *karma* with the present *karma*, let us take an example on a smaller time scale. When we eat something which is not suitable for us or we over-eat, we may suffer from indigestion. This is an immediate result of our *karma*. When we feel unwell, then we do further *karma* by curing ourselves. With appropriate medication and care, we succeed in curing ourselves. Thus, with our present *karma*, we have deleted the effect of the past *karma*. On the other hand, if we ignore our minor disorders and continue to do such actions, which enhance the ailment, gradually, it will acquire a serious dimension. In that case, to restore the equilibrium, we will have to take regular therapeutic measures for a long time. The situation may be reverse than in the above example. A person who makes a regular effort to be in harmony with space and time for good health and longevity will harvest the fruits of his/her positive actions or *karma*.

According to Caraka, **"There is no major action the fruits of which are not attained. The diseases caused by *karma* (of the past) neutralise the therapeutic measures and subside only on the destruction of these deeds"**[7]

The results of previous *karma* cannot be predetermined otherwise our present *karma* in terms of personal effort will lose its importance. In that case, all health care practices will lose their

7 *Caraka Saṃhitā*, *Śarīrasthānam*, I, 117

importance. Our will, determination, persistence and devotion to cure ourselves are very important. For example, if we have an ailment due to our previous *karma*, our present action of how we handle this ailment ultimately decides how much suffering we get from this ailment. Besides the appropriate treatment, our will, determination and persistence play an important part in healing. In other words, our present *karma* interferes with the past *karma* and it is the net result of the two, which is a determining factor of the course of healing. The present human action cannot be predicted as it depends upon the individual intellect (*buddhi*). It is not possible to predetermine the human action and therefore it is also not possible to predetermine any course of future ailments or diseases.

We may say that the minor ailments are the results of our immediate *karma* and in most cases, by taking immediate measures, we can restore health. Our negligence and an erroneous way of living generally cause many of the innate disorders (see Section III for details of different types of disorders). This latter means not to live according to our fundamental nature or *prakṛti* with which all of us are born due to the effect of our previous *karma*. It also includes not living in harmony with time and space. Gradually, we attain a state of imbalance that comes to surface one-day in the form of a serious innate disorder like diabetes, colitis, chronic aches and pains or a mental imbalance.

A big incurable disease may be the result of an extremely erroneous living style over a long period of time or an accumulated effect of the *karma* from the past lives. For example, when a baby is born with a big disease or a serious disease suddenly attacks a person despite a health-promoting holistic life style, the cause may be the accumulated *karma* of the past life or even lives.

Personal effort in terms of our present *karma* is important in case of all kinds of disorders. Our effort done with devotion, persistence, determination and intuitive wisdom will bear some fruits and accelerate the healing process. Even in case of the incurable disorders, all these efforts should be made to lessen the suffering and to attain good death. The term 'good death' may surprise many of you in the West as this concept is alien to the western mind and more so to the Western medical system.

In case of serious, incurable diseases, the role of spiritual therapy is very important to lessen the bad effect of the past *karma*.

Spiritual therapy also includes giving donations, doing good deeds in one way or the other planting healing trees, oblations and other similar acts with the wish of getting cured.

Training oneself with various yogic practices is an asset in life for maintaining good health and harmony. The utilization of all these to keep mental balance as well as for spiritual therapy is tremendous. These methods are not learnt in one day and when one is already sick, it is rather difficult to learn restraint, self-discipline etc. As the Chinese will put it- one does not make weapons when there is already a war.

Use of yogic practices in therapy and healing

Use of various yogic practices is done at diverse levels for therapy and healing. The whole process of awareness of body, self-discipline, self-restraint, yogic postures and breathing practices from the classical yoga has been adopted in Āyurveda. The yogic practices are extremely important for the care of the body, its maintenance and to have a radiant look. They play an important role in acquiring inner poise and harmony. Yogic practices are as important for the body as plaster for a brick wall, which renders strength, smoothness and beauty to it. A wall without plaster does not fall but is not protected and it tends to have a shorter life. It is easily affected by extreme weather conditions. It does not have a smooth look and is not pleasant to touch. Massaging the body may be equated to painting the plastered wall.

Yoga is a part of Āyurvedic therapy in all its dimensions–rational, mental and spiritual. It is a part of rational therapy when we cure various posture defects, aches and pains by yogic movements and postures. The yogic exercises are not mechanical and they demand our full concentration and obviously we mentally participate in our cure, which is the second dimension of the Āyurvedic therapy. From breathing and concentration practices, various healing methods are evolved which form the third dimension of the Āyurvedic therapy—the spiritual healing. Nevertheless, in most cases, it is not possible to cure oneself exclusively with yoga therapy, as we also need medication and nutrition therapy.

One must clearly understand that yoga and Āyurveda merge together because for both of them the well-being of the body is of prime importance. Āyurvedic practices like outer and inner cleaning of the body are also a part of yoga. Yoga has also some different cleaning practices than Āyurveda. The adepts of yoga are also aware of various other Āyurvedic health care practices and medicinal plants. Their bodies have to be in perfect equilibrium for attaining success in yogic postures and breathing practices. Patañjali has clearly stated that sickness is first of the thirteen major obstacles in the path of yoga (Part 1, Sūtras 30, 31; see Table 4).

SECTION V

Āyurvedic Yoga

What is Āyurvedic yoga?

I have coined this special term in order to be more specific about which aspect of Patañjali's yoga we are using and for what purpose. I also want to emphasise here that the Āyurvedic yoga I am going to describe here is fundamentally derived from Patañjali's eight-fold yoga. The basic purpose of Āyurvedic yoga is to maintain good health, physical and mental harmony and to have a feeling of well-being. It is by all this that we can succeed in warding off big ailments and diseases. The Āyurvedic yoga is essential for the adepts of the yoga for achieving *kaivalya* and for others for the purpose of acquiring peace and harmony in life. Body is the medium for *bhoga*—the sensuous joys on the one hand and medium for the yoga or spiritual liberation on the other hand. The Āyurvedic yoga described here is basically for the well-being of the body. I remind the reader once more that when I use the word body in the context of yoga, Āyurveda or Indian tradition in general, it is meant for the whole being and not just for the physical body without mind, intellect and soul.

Caraka says, **"Adherence to not discriminating between non-eternal (our physical self) and eternal (our soul) as well as wholesome and unwholesome is known as derangement of intellect as by nature the intellect sees rightly."**[1]

Patañjali's view is similar when he talks of *avidyā* or ignorance, which is the cause of afflictions. *Avidyā* is not to distinguish the eternal soul from the non-eternal body. In fact, when we bring our mind to stillness by hindering the chain of thoughts (Part I, Sūtra 2), the mind comes to the *Sattva* State (intellect or *Buddhi*) and this by nature has discriminative power and sees the right. In this state, we have the intuitive wisdom to know the details of our physical and mental self and tend to take the right decisions for our health as well as for our well-being in general. Caraka adds further that due to the derangement of intellect,

[1] *Caraka Saṃhitā, Śarīrasthānam,* I, 100.

mind looses its restraint and indulges in unwholesome sensuous pleasures, which obviously ruin the health. This leads to excess of *rajas* and *tamas* and lack of *sattva* leading to the derangement of memory.[2]

This section has five Chapters dealing with various aspects of Āyurvedic yoga. The first Chapter is about the initiation into Āyurvedic yoga with some simple practices. The second Chapter deals with some aspects of the purification of the body and mind for the purpose of good health, mental strength and well-being. The third Chapter deals with the *āsanas* (yogic postures) and *prāṇāyāma* and their practical importance for creating physical and mental equilibrium. The fourth Chapter is on prevention and cure of ailments and it deals with the factors like tension, stress, worries or other emotional burdens, which are the major causes of ailments and are generally ignored. The fifth and last Chapter deals with the 'living' element in the body explaining the subtle energy all of us have and how we can channelise this energy for our benefit.

All these five Chapters deal with the practical aspects of life and simple programmes are given for you to begin practising as you are proceeding further. The Āyurvedic yoga provides you the wisdom about life and various suggestions and practises for strengthening the body and the mind and developing courage and spiritual powers.

---

2 *Caraka Saṃhitā, Śarīrasthānam,* I, 101.

CHAPTER 1

Initiation into Āyurvedic Yoga

As you have seen from the fundamentals of Āyurveda, the states of body and mind are interrelated and interdependent. Imbalance of one of the humours leads also to change the mental state besides having other effects at the physical level. Similarly, our mental state can also cause an imbalance of the humours. For example, *vāta* disturbance will give rise to hectic and nervous mental state whereas a hectic and stressful state of mind will cause *vāta* imbalance in the body. *Pitta* disturbances may lead to an angry state of mind whereas anger may enhance *pitta*. *Kapha* dis-turbance can give depression and depression may cause an imbalance of *kapha*. Thus, for good health and harmony, the balance of three humours as well as equilibrium of the three states of mind is very essential. These three states of mind are *sattva*, *rajas* and *tamas*. I repeat again as a reminder:*sattva* is the inner stillness, peace and harmony, *rajas* represents activity, force, action and movement and *tamas* is that which restraints, hinders and obstructs motion. I call it the six-dimensional equilibrium in Āyurveda and I have described it in details in my recent Āyurveda book.[3]

The three out of five parts the Patañjali's eight-fold yoga, which are important in the present context, are forebearance, self-discipline and restraint. The values and practices they suggest are largely to bring inner peace and harmony as well as the humoral equilibrium for promoting strength and health. These practices and values are also a part of classical Āyurveda, which is the science of life and aims at human well being, health, promoting the quality of life and longevity. The idea is to develop control over one's desires and develop an ability to have the stillness of mind. It is the lack of control over oneself that leads to excess of *tamas* and *rajas* and diminishes *sattva*. According to Caraka, **"Perverted, negative and excessive use of sense objects, time and intellect is the three-fold cause of both psychic and somatic disorders. Both body and mind are the locations of disorders as well as of pleasure. The Self (soul) is devoid of disorders."[4].**

---

[3] For details, refer to my book, *Sixteen Minutes to a Better 9-to-5.*

[4] *Caraka Saṃhitā, Sūtrasthānam,* I, 54-56.

It is generally observed that yoga, particularly in the West, is mostly taught with an emphasis on postures (*āsanas*) and breathing exercises (*prāṇāyāma*). Āyurveda is normally limited to *vāta, pitta* and *kapha* and that too with a reductionist approach by ignoring the holistic aspect of the discipline. Yoga teachers often do not teach the purification of the mind in the yoga classes. **"The mind is purified by an attitude of friendship, compassion, satisfaction and indifference equally towards the sense objects giving rise to happiness, sorrow, virtue and non-virtue."** (Part 1, ***Sūtra*** 33). While teaching Āyurveda in the West, it is completely ignored that it is our state of mind which is the root cause of ailments and that the key to good health is to attain a mental state of satisfaction or *santoṣa* (see next Chapter for details). It is these basic values that I want to emphasise in the Āyurvedic yoga as they are mostly ignored in institutions. which aim to teach yoga for good health.

With a mental state of *santoṣa* or contentment, you will remain a *prasannacitta* person (that with a happy disposition). According to Āyurvedic sages, a happy disposition by itself is a major factor to prevent ailments. Lack of contentment gives rise to negative qualities like excessive desires, anger, greed and so on. In this world, there is no end to desires for material possessions as well as for sensuous fulfilment. Happiness lies within us; it is not a commercial commodity that can be bought. It is by constant practice of restraint that one can learn to control the mind from indulging into negative qualities. The breathing practices as well as the yogic postures help to develop a control over one's thought process. These practices are based on very sophisticated techniques where body controls the mind and mind controls the body. They both develop a dialogue. Gradually with constant practice, a complete mastery over one's thinking process is attained. The next step is to attain the capability to stop the thinking process. When this is attained, the mind acquires oneness with the soul (which is the cause of consciousness) instead of oneness with our sensuous self. When the mind remains in a normal state, it has a constant chain of thoughts with the information it is receiving from the senses, it identifies itself with our physical being. When we withdraw ourselves from the senses, reach a state of stillness and are successful in hindering the thinking process, our mind identifies itself with our soul (see Figure 11 on page 43). This is a state when the mind becomes capable of experiencing 'other reality' than the sensuous. The mind is bound by time as far as it identifies itself with our sensuous self, which is short-lived and destructible. But when it identifies with the eternal energy, it is no more time bound and is able to see the past, future, distant, hidden and minute aspects of reality. This is what we call also the intuitive wisdom, spiritual lucidity or spiritual power etc. Our purpose in Āyurvedic yoga is to develop this spiritual lucidity for the purpose of exploring our body and to develop intuitive knowledge. It is important to know about all those factors that directly or indirectly lead to bad health, in order to prevent ailments and to develop the ability to strengthen weak parts and healing ailing parts. It is also used to develop energy armour around us to save ourselves from bad events, ill thoughts or infections etc. and to acquire a beautiful radiant look.

Let us see how Caraka has put his views on the values described in Patañjali's yoga.

> **"The unwholesome action performed by one whose intellect, restraint and memory are deranged is known as intellectual error. It vitiates all the doṣas (humours). Propulsion of urges and their suppression, indulgence in exerting actions and excessive sexuality, hectic or delayed actions, wrong initiation of actions, disappearance of modesty and good conduct, rebuking the respected ones, knowingly using unwholesome things, use of factors which cause severe derangement of mind, movement in wrong place and time, friendship with the wicked, avoiding noble code of conduct described in the chapter of introductory description of the senses, envy, conceit, fear, anger, greed, ignorance, narcosis and confusion, troublesome actions taken under their spell, troublesome bodily actions and other such actions arising from *rajas* and *tamas* is said as the intellectual error by the nobles, which is the cause of diseases."[5]**

In my opinion, the basic values of the Yoga and Āyurveda should be taught to those who come to seek help of yoga for a healthy living. As far as health is concerned, yoga without the basics of Āyurveda will not be completely beneficial and of course

---

5. *Caraka Saṃhitā, Śarīrasthānam,* I, 102-108. For the 'use of senses', refer to *Sūtrasthānam,* I, 54 and also see my book, *Āyurveda, A Way of Life,* Chapter 8.

yogic values, postures etc. are an important part of the Āyurvedic therapy. Thus, I have founded Āyurvedic yoga and given the programmes in such a way that you assimilate this wisdom in its multiple dimensions and make it a way of life. In these programmes, you will learn how to heal and cure certain ailments and get rid of some chronic and nagging health problems with the combination of Āyurvedic and yogic methods. In addition, I will also provide concise methods to get rid of stress and enhance concentration and memory. There will be a gradual awareness of all the body parts, inner functions, importance of inner cleanliness etc. finally leading to the wisdom about the subtle body, which is the energy body that lies in our physical body. The aim of this is prevention and healing of the ailments. As is evident, all this programme depends upon the fundamental idea of control of the mind, which we will achieve through yogic exercises, postures, breathing practices and simple exercises of concentration based upon Patañjali's yogic principles. All this is to say that most of the yogic practices you are usually learning in yoga schools are actually the means to achieve something and they are not the end by themselves.

The following programmes, which will run throughout this Section of the book, are not in the form of the yogic sessions of one hour daily or so. They will involve your life situations in general and are also meant to help you incorporate the basic values of yoga and Āyurveda in your daily life with the help of simple, sometimes funny exercises.

Programme number one

In this programme, we will take up some simple yogic thoughts, exercises and postures to make you aware of the process of self-control and concentration. I will also explain how all this works scientifically.

Exercise number 1: *Following yourself*

(a) **A rhythmic walk:** You may do this exercise anywhere and any time. In fact, try to make it a habit. It involves simply checking yourself how you sit or walk or talk. It is like mirroring your image in your mind. Take a small walk after dinner, preferably alone, if not, stay quiet. Inhale in first two steps and exhale in the next two. You may make your steps longer or shorter according to your breathing capacity. If you repeat this exercise for a few days, you will realise that automatically you will be walking in an aware manner and your walking and breathing will co-ordinate with each other.

(b) **Scanning your body:** While you are sitting, it may be at work or at home or sitting just for relaxation to read something, or sitting to eat your meal and so on, let yourself loose. Make a quick journey of your whole body with your thoughts. Begin from the area near your heart and from this point, scan the head region, then both your arms simultaneously up to the extremities (hands) and then the central part up to the base of your body from where you can simultaneously follow both your legs up to your feet. With a little practice, all this can be done in the duration of one deep breath. Keep practising until you achieve this. Then make it a habit to do this 'scanning process' whenever you can during the day. Specially before meals or before beginning some important work or before beginning to drive and so on. The idea is to train you to be with yourself and in all your actions your whole being should be present. That means you are not mechanically performing your actions and activities.

(c) **Reverting to your thoughts:** This is the last part of this series and it involves breaking your thought process and reverting to your thoughts and trying to recall what you were thinking during the last few minutes. It is not to recall your thoughts in a gross manner but in fine details. It is kind of 'catching yourself' and 'replaying' what was going on a few minutes ago. This exercise will make you conscious how the chain of thoughts works with association. It will also help you to develop concentration and enhance memory.

Exercise number 2: *Checking yourself*

This exercise involves checking your body to see if all parts are in a state of relaxation. It is an extremely important exercise as most of us store tension in one part or the other. This becomes a part of us and we do not even notice it. It comes to the surface only when this particular part of our body begins to protest. This protest surfaces in the form of pain or stiffness. Even at that stage, most of us do not realise the real cause behind it. If we keep scrutinising our bodies, then we can get rid of the pain not yet come.

Let me give you some simple examples of this tension I am talking about. At the moment, I am sitting in front of the computer and writing this book. At times, I have to stop for a while and think about the next idea or the way a sentence should be formulated and so on. But during this time, my wrists, hands and fingers stay in a state of tension waiting for the next order. What is better for me is to check myself and release this tension with a deep breath from time to time. Along with this, I should check the following: my sitting posture, my shoulders, backbone etc. which are in a 'ready to do' state. Therefore it is better that during my work, let us say after each paragraph, I relax for 2 or three breaths and 'check myself' by 'following my body' as has been described above.

I will state few more examples in this connection. People who have plenty of varied things to do and during this process they have to sit, stand and walk many times, they tend to store tension in their legs and more so if their fundamental nature is *vāta*. In this case, concentrate on the lower part of the back, which supplies energy to the legs. People who sit a lot and do desk work generally get tension in the abdomen and have often *pitta* disturbances. Right shoulder tension is another very common phenomenon. In some cases, both the shoulders and neck tend to be in the state of tension. There are others who keep their forehead frowned or store tension in the muscles around their mouth. Like a policeman who controls the traffic for a smooth flow, you may keep a check on your various body parts. It is just a habit you have to develop and later you will automatically begin to keep a watch on yourself.

Exercise number 3: *Expanding yourself in space*

The body is made of five fundamental elements one of which is ether. Ether along with air makes one of the three major vital forces or humours- the *vāta*. Ether is space in practical sense and it has multiple facets at various dimensions of reality. But in the present context, what I want to convey in very simple words is that if we limit ourselves too much in space, we may face health problems. Going for a walk is not only important for a physical exercise but also for the intake of the cosmic energy which is ether. It is very common these days that people buy different equipments for exercising in their apartments. My suggestion is that you should try to expand yourself in space and get out of the houses and apartments as much as possible. Some people gain weight and they claim that they have plenty of physical activities in their homes and despite that, they put on weight. Physical exercise in a limited space has less effect than when your activity is carried on in bigger areas.

By sitting too much, we shrink the internal space of our body and harm ourselves in several ways. Therefore, do the stretching exercises from time to time even if you have to do long hours of work that involves sitting at one place. Supposing you are in a meeting that lasts many hours and it is not possible to do the stretching exercises. At least move your abdominal muscles up and down and in and out.

Some stretching exercises

1. Stretch both your arms at the back, cross the fingers of both your hands and stretch them as far back as possible. In this process, both your shoulders will bend backward (Figure 15). While in this posture, try to move your arms in left and right directions.
2. In a similar manner, stretch forward and this time push few times up and down (Figure 16).
3. Stretch upward in a similar manner with clasped hands. Your head will be between your two arms. Make circular movements 2-3 times clockwise and then anti-clockwise (Figure 17). These movements should be done from the waist and not from the lower part of the back. Do the movements slowly so that all your back and neck muscles are revitalised with this exercise. Leave a gap of 3-4 breaths between the clockwise and anticlockwise movements.
4. Bend backward and forward with the clasped hands and upwards stretched arms (Figure 18, 19).

Exercise number 4: *Keeping the mental equilibrium*

To keep the mental equilibrium, you should bring *sattva* in your everyday life that is generally lacking in daily routine. Our lives are mostly dominated by *rajas* and *tamas.* The above-described exercises with breathing help bring some stillness in the modern

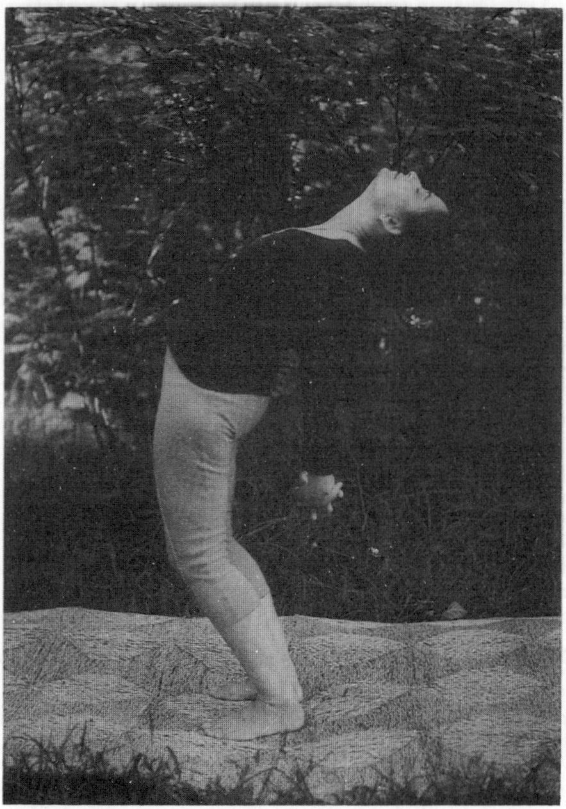

Figure 15. Backward stretching exercise

life, which is hectic and full of activities. Everyday, you should take a few minutes to review your daily activities and see if you had feelings of jealousy, competition, anger, possessiveness or other similar feelings, which hinder growth and are *tāmasic*. Exercise your mind by convincing yourself that these ill feelings are going to do you harm ultimately and they are not going to solve any problem. You have to make a constant and persistent effort. To help yourself in this effort, repeat one word of your liking hundred and one times. You may choose OṂ, which is the symbol of cosmic energy. As you pronounce the word once, the image of the number should appear between your eyebrows. Your eyes should remain closed. This exercise will gradually purify your

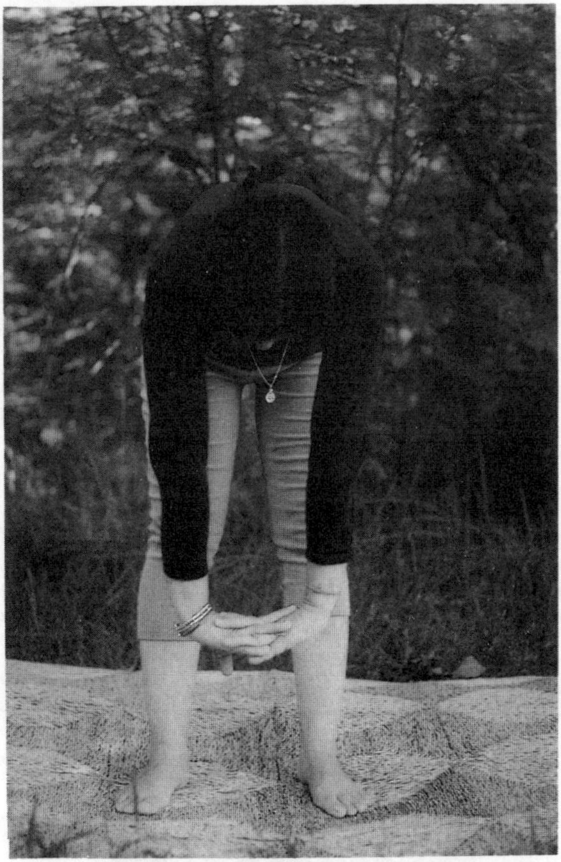

Figure 16. Forward stretching exercise.

mind from ill feelings and will provide you spiritual strength.

Programme number two

In this programme, we will take four different yogic postures or *āsanas* of a series that involves mainly lifting your leg or legs up while in supine position and while lying down on your stomach. They are called *Uttānapāda āsanas. Uttāna* means raising and *pāda* means limb (leg). You will be initiated into these four *āsanas* but in the beginning, they will be more like a slow exercise. These will be retaken later in the book and they will help you to

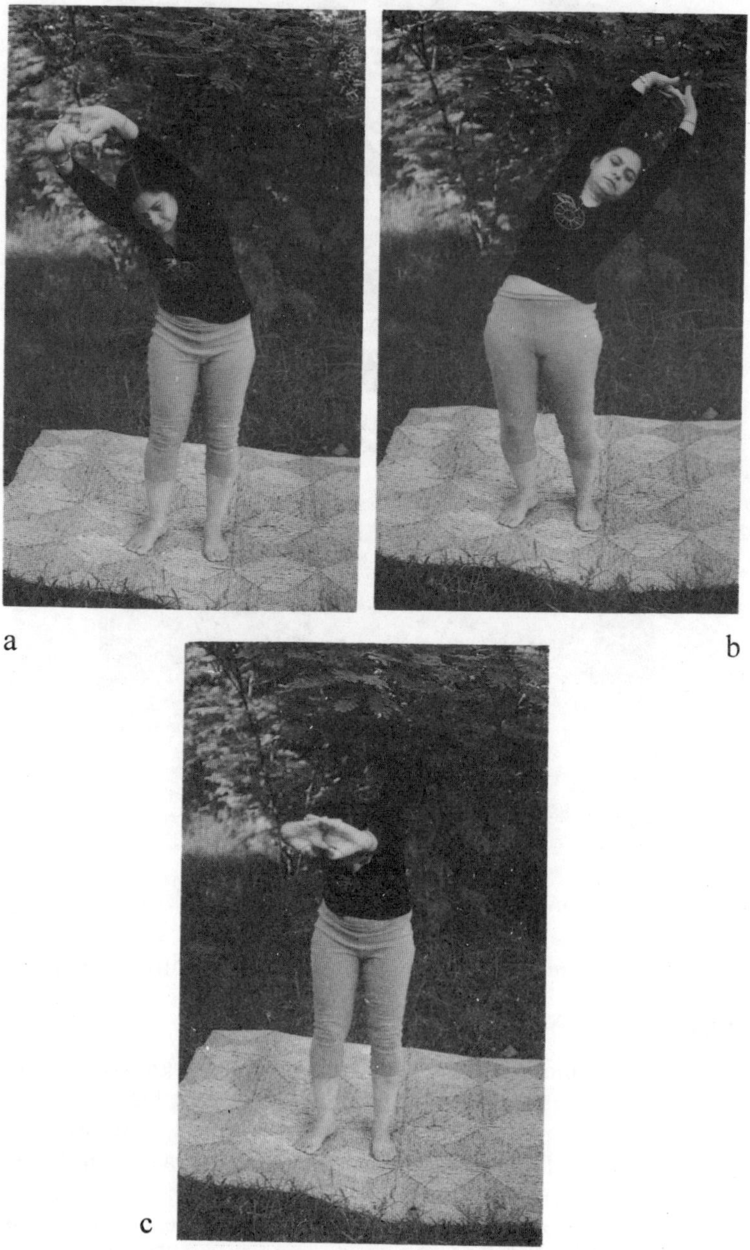

a b c

Figure 17, a to c. Round movements with upward stretching.

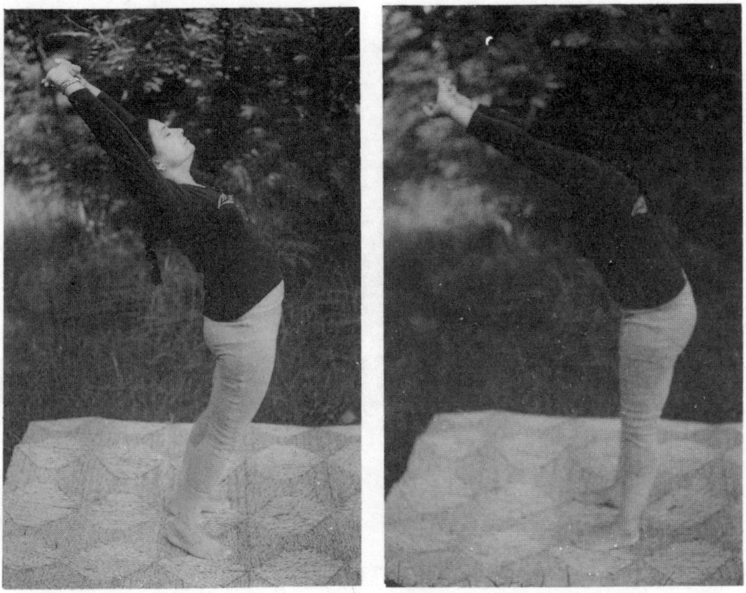

Figures 18 & 19. Backward and forward stretching with upward stretched arms.

understand what an *āsana* actually is and how it differs from an exercise.

Following are the four different *uttānapāda āsanas*:

1. Lie down on your back with your legs nearly thirty centimetre apart from each other and your arms stretched out. Make yourself at ease and let yourself loose. Breathe deeply and in a rhythmical manner. Gradually lift up your left leg while you inhale. Do not bend your knee in this process and the force of lifting up should come from your pelvic region (Figure 20). Lift up as much as possible without forcing yourself. If you force yourself, your lifted leg will start trembling. Hold your breath and keep the leg still in the upward position for a few seconds. Bring the leg down gradually while you are exhaling. Rest for two or three breaths and then do the same exercise with your right leg. Repeat this five to ten times.

   While doing this exercise, you should pay attention to two major things: 1) Your breathing should co-ordinate with

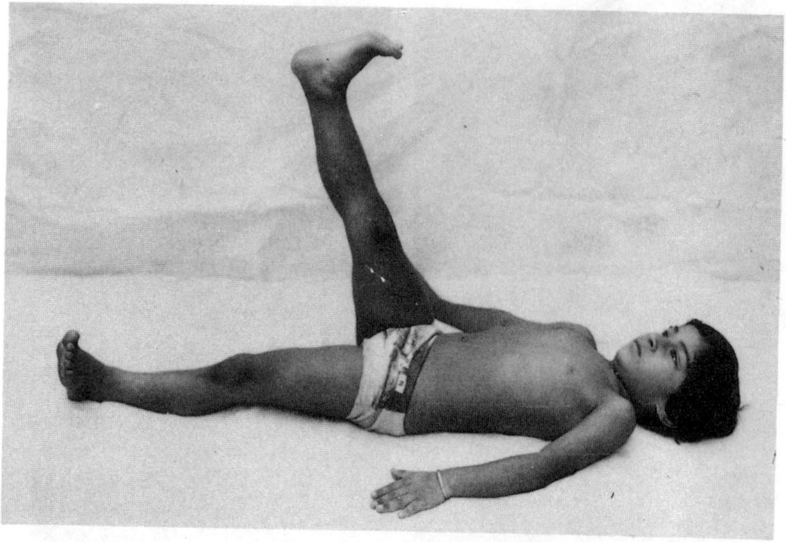

Figure 20. *Uttānapāda āsana* 1, lifting one leg at a time while lying on the back.

your movements and both should be gradual and rhythmical. 2) You should lift your leg a little higher each time but stop before you get any tension in your muscles. You will realise that very gradually, your capacity to raise the leg higher will enhance.

2. This exercise involves lifting both the legs together. For this, you lie down on your back but this time your feet should be close together. The rest of the process is the same except that you are lifting both your legs with the feet joined together (Figure 21). Co-ordinate the breathing in similar manner as described above.

3-4. These exercises are done in the similar manner as above but by lying down on your stomach (Figures 22 & 23).

Later in the book, I will talk about the concept of an *āsana* and how these exercises described here are perfected to make a yogic posture. But before that in the next chapter, we will take up the theme of purification of body and mind leading to self-discipline and restraint. Without these basic requirements, it is not possible to attain success in yoga *āsanas* and *prāṇāyāma*.

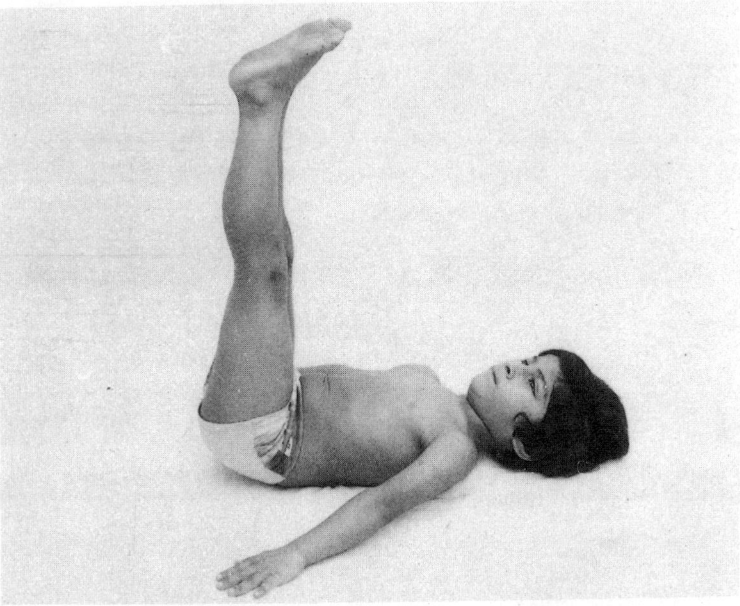

Figure 21. *Uttānapāda āsana* 2, lifting two legs together while lying on the back.

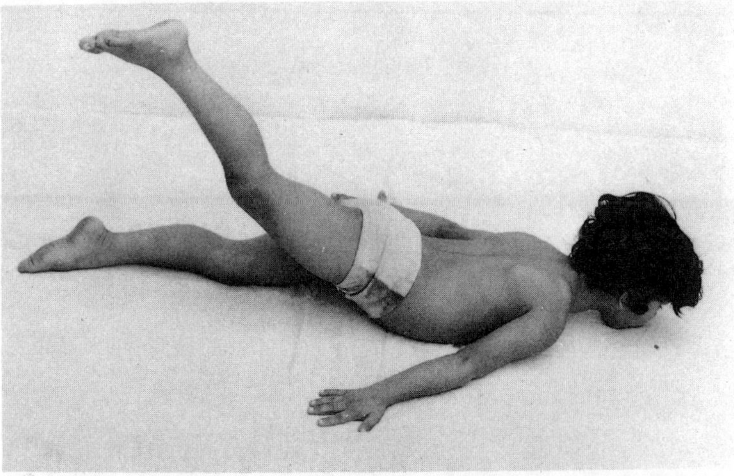

Figure 22. *Uttānapāda āsana* 3, lifting one leg at a time while lying on the abdomen.

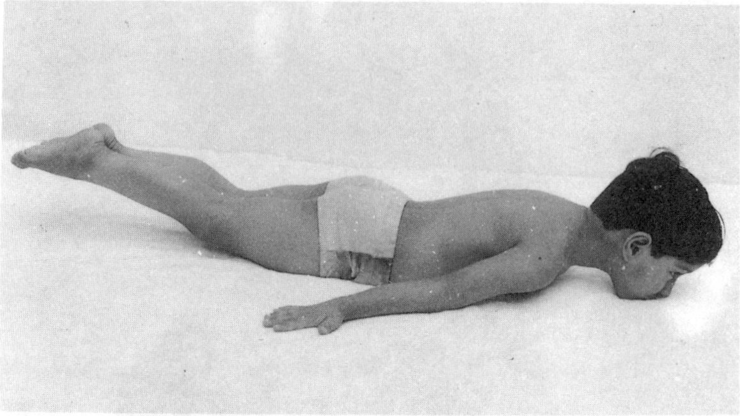

Figure 23. *Uttānapāda āsana* 4, lifting both the legs together while lying on the abdomen.

CHAPTER 2

Purification of the Body and the Mind

Inter-relationship of the body and the mind

For both yoga and Āyurveda, the purification at different levels is of primary importance. It is by purification that one can get the physical and mental strength to achieve the aim of yoga. In Āyurveda, for maintaining equilibrium of the humours, the inner and outer purification practices are extremely important (see Section III for details). For therapeutic purposes, very highly specialised purification practices are done. Dirt at the physical level disturbs also the mind and when the mind is cluttered with negative thoughts, the process of accumulation of dirt at the physiological level also begins. Thus, the purification of both body and mind is essential for keeping good health, and physical and mental strength, which may be used for the purpose of achieving the aim of yoga or for sensuous fulfilment or material gains.

Before I proceed further, let me explain my above statement with some examples. Supposing you are suffering from constipation. The reason for your constipation may be your negligence of taking appropriate diet and lack of movements. Let us say that you eat too much bread, cheese, meat, biscuits etc. and take less vegetables, soups and salads. On the top of it, you have to sit for hours to finish an assignment. Thus, you get constipation purely due to not paying attention. This is accumulation of dirt in your body. The dirt inside at a high temperature ferments and produces stink which destroys the inner environment of your body. This will give you a feeling of discomfort, bad sleep or disturbing dreams. All this will make you nervous and negative thoughts will begin entering your mind. You may get easily irritated, hectic in your mannerisms and may get a state of confusion in your mind. If you do not cure the root cause of all these problems and purify yourself, first of all at physical level, the problems may further complicate. For example, in a state of nervousness and confusion, you may make more mistakes in your work and that may lead to tension and thus cause further constipation and allied problems to a greater degree.

Let us take an example of a case where the problems begin at the mental level. You are preparing for a job interview and you think that you are the appropriate person to get this job. You are very hopeful and you make best of your efforts to get this job. But you do not get this job and somebody else who you think is less competent, gets this job. You are over-powered by the feelings of jealousy, competition and dejection. All these *tamasic* thoughts give you digestive disorders. You feel uncomfortable after eating and get distension. That irritates you further as you are already in an unhappy mental state. The irritation further complicates your digestive problems. Thus, contrary to the above situation, in this case you need to purify your mind to get rid of the root cause of your physical discomfort.

By giving above examples, I want to make you aware of how the holistic concepts of yoga and Āyurveda look at the relationship of body and mind and how you can learn to steer one with the other. Basically, it is the understanding of these problems which is essential. Taking the first example, if you remain unaware that your problem of bad dreams originated from constipation, you would not be able to cure yourself though the treatment is extremely simple. It will be still more unfortunate if you visit a non-holistic (coined term) physician who would prescribe some tranquillisers for you. By this treatment, you will start a series of events in your body, which will take you away from the fundamental equilibrium essential for health. A similar thing can happen in the second example if you do not go to an appropriate physician to get treatment for your stomach problems.

The body-mind interaction is at diverse levels of our being and I will try to elucidate how you can learn to look at the problems from the holistic point of view at different levels of your existence and treat yourself with very simple yogic and Āyurvedic methods.

Interdependence of the body and the mind

The process of cleaning the body with Āyurvedic *pañcakarma* practices is not limited to the body cleaning. It also begins to clean your mind. This is the experience I have gathered over the years and have had some amazing case studies. With massages, purging, fomentation, enema etc., not only the *malas* (dirts) of the body come out, but it also touches the psyche of the person undergoing this treatment. People are surprised at their own behaviour and at times they do not know how to handle it. When they are told about this fact that their mind is getting cleaned with the body, they are reassured. There are persons who cannot face themselves and end up turning aggressive to me. In that situation also, as a therapist, I have to have patience and compassion to make them understand the real problem and to assure them that they are getting cured.

In fact, it is not only the process itself which makes them have a search within. If they go to a *pañcakarma* clinic and let them be handled by paramedical staff and let others massage them and so on, I do not think that the purification of their mind will happen in the similar manner. There are two principal factors that play a major role in this purification process. One is the fact that they are completely away from their own environment and are in a far away land. Second and the major factor is that it is probably the first time in their lives that they have taken so much time to work on their bodies. The process of mechanical living governed by the head, breaks down and their bodies and minds acquire a friendly and communicative relationship with each other. The fact of 'being with themselves', probably first time in their lives initiate them to have a journey within themselves. Let me quote below an example so that you can better comprehend my point.

This is a young woman who met me in Autumn in one of my seminars. She purchased from me a rejuvenating product and she booked a cure course with me here in India in the following winter. She had told me that she was buying that product for her mother who was very sick and weak. She was joining a small group of 4 persons in India after two months of this incident. After first few days of the cleaning practices, she showed a very aggressive behaviour and then suddenly she was over-powered by aches in her whole body, which lasted two days. She turned very docile afterwards probably due to the care she received at the time when she was unwell. I always spend some private time with each student and she was with me in this session. She told me that she was feeling like crying and tears were flowing for hours from her eyes. She felt that she had no control over herself. I explained to her that it was probably some accumulated pain that was finding an outlet. Amazingly she told me that her mother had died in May and probably that was the reason. Remember that this person had bought a product from me in November for her mother who had already died in May. Anyway, at last she was able to accept this death and could cry over it.

The blood purifying substances, which are supposed to detoxify the blood, so to say, have also amazing results on one's psyche. These substances are supposed to detoxify the whole body, not only the organisms, which are involved in the blood cells formation. These substances act on liver, throw out excess of heat from the body through faeces, urine and sweat and remove the bad smell from the body. I believe that each cell of our body is a cosmos by itself and it is capable of retaining information in the form of memory and also inter-communicating at a subtle level (that means more than just biological exchange). In that light, I further expand this theory by adding that blood goes to each and every part of the body and also to our brain. It is very likely that after getting detoxified, the blood has a pacifying effect on our brain cells and their inter-communication changes. In a way, they enhance the brain efficiency. I do not mean here that they enhance brain efficiency in the sense of promoting memory or power of creativity. For that we have another series of products in Āyurveda. What I mean to say here is that they enhance brain efficiency in terms of time. That means that some suppressed memories, emotions, experiences etc. are revoked. Thus, the blood purifying substances also purify our mind from the past afflictions or *kleśas*. We need to do more research in this direction and our organisation will continue to keep further records of these effects.

Various aspects of physical purification

A very simple purification practice we do everyday is taking a bath or a shower. The water you pour on yourself not only washes off the dirt, sweat and smell from your body, it also gives freshness and comfort to your mind. A kind of dullness persists if we start our day without a shower. Warm or hot bath or shower helps bring *vāta* and *kapha* in equilibrium. A cold bath brings *pitta* in equilibrium. Immediately after bath, one is able to concentrate better. A kind of calmness persists for a while and it is easy to get a thought-free mind immediately after a bath.

In various bodies of yogic literature as well as in numerous present day schools of yogic tradition, a large number of methods to do inner cleansing of the body are prescribed. However, my aim is not to confuse you with numerous methods but rather be extremely precise and give only those methods which can be used in our times with facility keeping in view the constraints of time in modern day life. In Section III, I have given briefly the Āyurvedic purification practices. These practices should be done twice a year at the end of two principal seasons. I have made this programme fairly simple and feasible in my book, *Sixteen Minutes to a better 9-to5.* You can do the purification practices on your own along with a programme for the practices which should be done prior to the purification practices. However, some practical training with a good teacher is recommended and after that you can benefit from this wisdom on your own the rest of your life. In this programme, I have also given some simple yogic practices of purification and have given simplified methods for cleaning the head region.

It is absolutely essential for the practice of *yogāsanas* and *prāṇāyāma* to have a clear nasal passage and a clean stomach and intestines. Since in our times, atmospheric pollution is tremendous, I would suggest that you should do the practice of *jalaneti* once a week. Food and water are also polluted, and in fact, we do not know what we are eating and drinking these days. Generally the ill effects of the chemicals we are subjected to are known much later and by that time we have consumed them for years. Therefore, I suggest that you should do the yogic practice of *jaladhauti* once a week. I will describe below briefly these two practices but once again I say that you should learn initially from a teacher- specially the *jalaneti.*

Jalaneti

This practice involves putting water from one nasal passage and taking it out from the other. This practice clears the nasal passages and makes it possible to have an unhindered flow of *prāṇa* energy. It also makes the nasal passage resistant to infections and irritations. It will prove specially beneficial to those who get frequent attacks of cold, hay fever, headaches, specially migraines. It enhances the sense of smell and gives a general feeling of well-being.

For doing this practice, you need a *neti* pot. It is a small pot with a nozzle, which is generally made of brass. In Europe, they are made of clay or glass. Fill the pot with hot water- little less hot than what you will use to take a shower. Hold the pot in your right hand. Tilt your head slightly backwards and then on the left side but in a little forward direction. Now open your mouth and breathe freely from it. Let yourself loose and be in a completely relaxed position. Insert the nozzle of the pot into your right nostril and tilt the pot gently. Let the water enter into your right nostril and come out from the left (Figure 24). Normally, if the nasal passage is clear, the water should flow smoothly. Pour the water until the pot is empty. If the nasal passage is obstructed, you might have to stop in between and blow your nose strongly. This practice activates the nasal passage and salivary glands. You will have to spit, blow your nose and some water may come out of your eyes too. Repeat the above practice by inserting water from your left nostril.

Note: There are several versions of the neti for the nasal passage but this is a simple one. Some schools recommend to add salt in the water. Since some of you may get irritation from salt, it is better not to take it. In any case, sea salt, which is generally available in the world, may be too strong for this purpose. Add a pinch of rock salt. Take drinking water for this purpose if tap water in your area is not potable or contains chlorine.

Jaladhauti

This practice consists of drinking about 1/2 to 1 litre of slightly salted water after getting up in the morning and vomiting it out after about 10 minutes. Bend down at 45° angle and tickle your throat to throw out the water (Figure 25). Angle of the body is very important when you throw out. Do not bend down more than that. If you have difficulty in taking out the water, drink a little more next time.

How rapidly and easily one is able to vomit the water depends upon the individual constitution or *prakṛti.* People with *kapha* constitution can throw out the water easily, the *pitta* constitution comes in the middle and in case of those with *vāta* constitution, the water is quickly absorbed by the body and they may have difficulties. All the water may not come out at once and you may have to retry. It is good to have four or five impulses for throwing out water. The number of impulses should never be more than eight.

In a healthy person, the thrown out water is clear and tasteless. If your *vāta* is vitiated, you may have great difficulty in throwing

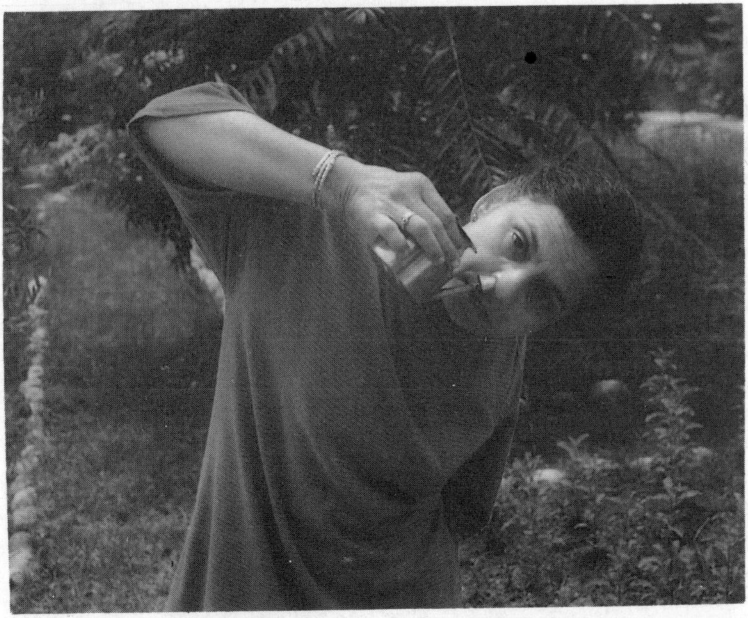

Figure 24. Practice of *Jalaneti.*

out the water. Sour or bitter taste indicates *pitta* vitiation. Foamy, whitish and slimy water indicates *kapha* vitiation. If undigested food comes out from the night before, you need to pay attention to this problem. In Āyurvedic terminology, this is called *amādoṣa.* The digestive fire is not strong enough to digest the food properly and undigested food remains in the stomach. The condition of *amādoṣa* may give rise to ailments like distension, gastritis, malabsorption of the nutrients, food poisoning etc. In fact, the undigested food rots and ferments in the body and causes infinite number of troubles. Thus, *jaladhauti* should also serve for you as a diagnostic practice. In case of *amādoṣa,* take the products which enhance the digestive fire (examples; ginger, pepper, ajwāin, dill seeds, cumin etc.). If the problem still persists, consult a holistic physician.

Mental purification

According to Patañjali, mental purification is essential to get rid of the afflictions, which are due to the desires for worldly

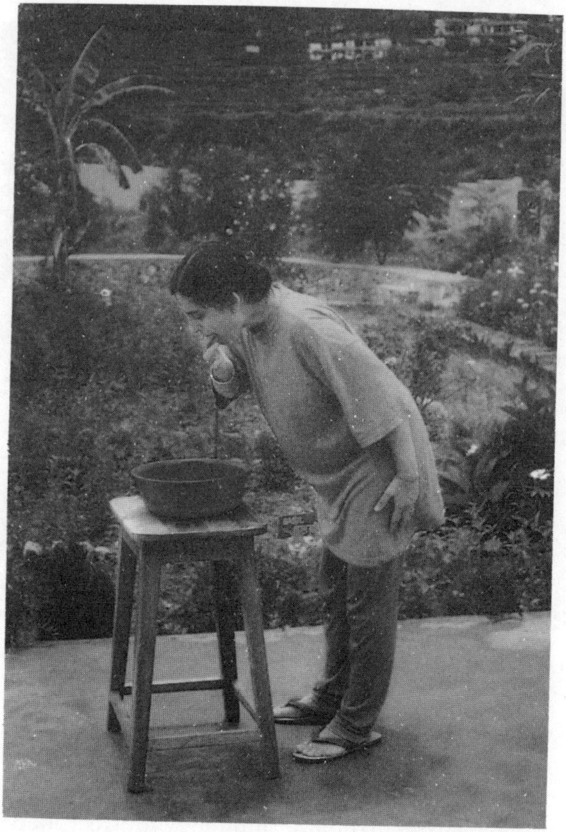

Figure 25. Practice of *Jaladhauti.*

pleasures. It is to achieve a mental state with a sense of satisfaction. When this state is achieved, one is able to experience inner joy and a steady state of mind. This state of mind is required for the subjugation of the senses for the purpose of yoga. After one has control over one's senses, one is able to realise the ultimate reality, the soul, which is the real self of an individual (Part I, Sūtra 41-42). Let us see which way all this is applied to Āyurvedic yoga to achieve good health and human well-being.

I have mentioned above the problem of *amādoṣa.* Let me quote here what Caraka writes about the causes of this disorder.

"...use of foods which are heavy, disliked, distending, burning, unclean, antagonistic and taken untimely. Other factors which also cause *amādoṣa* are the mental afflictions with psychic emotions such as passion, anger, greed, confusion, envy, bashfulness, grief, conceit, excitement and fear."[6]

When yoga and Āyurveda are taught in foreign countries or at a commercial level in India, generally these values are not talked about. However, in both disciplines, the sages talked extensively and demonstrated how they were of prime importance to achieve good health as well as stillness of mind for the purpose of achieving the aim of yoga.

Thus, we see that for good health and longevity, it is extremely essential to have control over one's emotions and develop the ability to control one's senses. Yoga provides us with various techniques to learn to do that. Both in yoga and Āyurveda, an emphasis is laid on *sattva* qualities and we have discussed this subject in the earlier part of this book. Let us take this theme in detail and explore about the *sattvic* values like truth, beauty, goodness, equilibrium, stillness etc. We can get over the *rajas* and *tamas* states of mind, which are predominant in our modern day life and cure many physical and mental ailments with sattvic values.

Our daily lives are generally full of activities and are quite hectic. We all have to run around and work for our living. We have to build the houses we live in, we have to organise to nourish ourselves and so on. All these are *rajas* activities. But these are not purely *rajas* activities, they are mixed with *tamas.* Many of us have to tell lies in our respective jobs. Directly or indirectly, all of us participate in killing and paining because of the use of so many pesticides. Besides that, many people eat meat and are directly involved in killing and paining. *Sattva* is lacking. After a hectic day, most people have a hectic evening of leisure with various activities for entertaining them. Then the night falls, it is time to rest and many want to close their eye and want to sleep very quickly so that they can have another hectic day after it. And the life goes on like that. There is a lack of stillness and inner peace, there are no sattvic actions.

---

6 *Caraka Saṃhitā, Vimānasthānam,* II, 8.

In former times, people had some sattvic activities because of several rituals in life. With the rituals like religious ceremonies or going to the church on Sunday, they were at least made conscious that there is a need to find inner peace and to develop harmony with cosmos or God which is a bigger power than what is visible with the senses. Then there were rituals observed at different stages of life; there were ceremonies performed which were directly or indirectly associated with spirituality and there were different ways of showing one's gratitude to nature, God or cosmos. For example, people said little prayers before their meals, before going to bed, before beginning a new task and so on. All this has slowly vanished specially from the metropolitan way of living and we are left with *rajas* and *tamas*. When the balance in the major three forces is lost and the *rajas* predominates overwhelmingly, there is a reaction to it and things may fall back in another extreme which is also not good for the well-being of the society. We should make every effort to bring in *sattva* in our lives so that the health of the society as well as of individuals can be maintained. Let us reflect a little on the factors which take us away from *sattva* and how we can lessen them or eradicate them. Caraka has described a *sattva* dominating person as follows:

> **"The persons having dominating *sattva* are endowed with memory, devotion, are grateful, learned, pure, courageous, skilful, resolute, fighting in battles with prowess, free from anxiety, having well directed and serious intellect and activities and are engaged in virtuous acts."[7]**

The anti-*sattva* seed: *Asantoṣa* or lack of contentment

Santoṣa in Sanskrit means the sense of satisfaction or contentment. This seems to be lacking in modern times. Contentment is an attitude of mind which people seem to have lost. There is a constant sense of dissatisfaction, which leads to *lobha* or greed. The Sanskrit word *lobha* means actually more than greed; it is not only to have the desire to possess what belongs to others or what we do not have, but also the desire to have more and more. The state of satisfaction should be maintained with a constant effort. Our mind has tremendous power and faculties. It goes on and

[7] *Caraka Saṃhitā, Vimānasthānam*, VIII, 110

on with new things in order to utilise its potentials. It is with our *buddhi* (intellect, sense to discriminate) that we have to direct its potentials. *Buddhi* is the *sattva* element of our being. If you wish to visualise in a diagrammatic form, *buddhi's* place is somewhere between soul and mind. When the mind acquires a state of stillness, it identifies itself with the soul and that is the state of mind during meditation. However the journey of mind to the soul requires tremendous amount of effort and time for an adept of yoga and all the four parts of Patañjali's *Yogasūtras* are about it. The domain of *buddhi* lies between the journey of the mind to the soul. When we temporarily acquire stillness of mind to concentrate on something particular or to do something precise and specific, we are already on that way and our mind stops to get cluttered with the senses and gets enlightened from the soul. That is what the *buddhi* is. The *buddhi* has different levels depending upon how far it is from the senses in its journey towards the soul or how close it is to the soul. An adept of yoga has to cross all these stages of *buddhi* to attain a complete oneness with the soul (see Part IV, Sūtra 26). But in the context of Āyurvedic yoga, for the well-being of our worldly existence, we have to learn to utilise our *buddhi* to control our mind. Recall the citation given in Section I of this book. The sages of Upaniṣads said that body is like a chariot, soul is the owner, *buddhi* or intellect is the driver, mind plays the part of reins and senses are horses while the world is the arena for all this. What I mean to say in the present context is that with the ability and capability of the driver (*buddhi*), we can use the reins of the chariot in such a way that it stays on the road and does not go in the mud. This way, both the driver and the chariot are safe and can enjoy the beauty of the world. Patañjali's yogī's aim is of course to take the owner to the destination.

The essence of all this detailed description is that we should learn to live at a little higher level than that of the senses and the mind and should use our *buddhi* to achieve a state of contentment or *santoṣa*. For living at the level of *buddhi*, we need inner stillness and I am describing many simple methods to achieve that in this part of the book. Initiation for that has been already given in the programmes of the last chapter. After learning to follow and check your mental activity, you will learn yogic *āsanas*, *prāṇāyāma* and other exercises for mental training in the next chapter.

I will elaborate here a little more on how *asantoṣa* or lack of contentment sows the seeds for other evils and how we get trapped into so many *kleśas* or afflictions. We lose our peace of mind and inner stillness and in these conditions we cannot also reach the state of *buddhi.* I have already talked about *lobha,* which comes out of lack of contentment. Let me elaborate this a little more and show you how at diverse levels *lobha* causes us mental and physical afflictions.

Let us take a simple and basic fact for our survival—the food. Food is life and also a cause of enjoyment as it fulfils the senses. I have described details of Āyurvedic nutrition in my Āyurveda books. Despite all these good qualities, due to *lobha,* we can turn the food into *kleśa* rather than pleasure. Or in other words we can say, it leads ultimately to *kleśa.* People initially eat to their satisfaction at the physiological level (2/3 of the stomach full, instructs Āyurveda). But due to *lobha,* they eat more than that and make themselves 'full'. If they do that everyday, it leads to the imbalance of all the humours giving rise to many ailments. Many get also over-weight and then they look for various methods to get rid of that. How ironical!

Lobha predominates in getting material gains, means of comfort, fame and so on. People seem to be never satisfied with what they have. In this process, they over-work, get nervous, get sleep problems and hundreds of other minor disorders. Many of them regret that they have time for nothing but work. But to get more time for themselves and their loved ones, they are not prepared to sacrifice a part of their enormous gains. The *lobha* is that they want to eat their cake and have it too. They want to have both- 'this' and 'that' simultaneously. There are limitations in life in terms of time, space and energy. Such people part from this world with the sense of *asantoṣa* or dissatisfaction.

Asantoṣa also leads to envy, jealousy, competition, anger and confusion. All this leads to a state of unhappiness and this latter gives rise to different ailments and disorders, thus giving rise to more *kleśas.* We get trapped in the vicious cycle and lose all pleasures of life. If we inculcate in ourselves the sense of being contented and satisfied then comes to us the wisdom to control all these emotions. Some say that a sense of contentment will lead to a dull and non-progressive attitude. Well, it depends on what one implies by progress. If the progress has to be at the cost of our health and entails mental pain, we will have to reconsider it. Besides, *santoṣa* is not at all anti-progress as far as the intellect, science, technology and so on are considered. It is our excessive involvement with the work, people, worldly objects and self-centred aims that bring the state of *asantoṣa.* In fact, Caraka talks again and again of 'intellectual error' that means in a sense any inventions, discoveries or decisions that ultimately lead to non-holistic and finally non-beneficial ends.

Another level of *asantoṣa* is in human relationships, particularly man-woman relationship. People want more and more from others, become possessive, overly attached and at times obsessed with the other human being. They are not satisfied with what others can give them of their time and energy and this state of *asantoṣa* leads to frictions and frustrations. In the relationship of couples, many hanker after more and more joy and instead of working hard on one relationship and making it more profound and beautiful, they change partners or have relationship on the sly with another woman or man. Generally, human beings are not grateful if they have a good partner. The reason for *asantoṣa* is also that the relationships are not seen at a spiritual or holistic level but like a consumer's item. This latter aspect is noticed when a couple lives long with each other, happy together and fulfilled and one of them falls sick or dies, he/she looks for a new partner in no time. It happens very often in the West that after 30, 40 or 50 years of companionship, when one is left alone, the other seeks a replacement in no time. This kind of attitude only leads to frustration and unhappiness. You should think with gratefulness the good and harmonious time you have had with one particular person and also think of all those who are not fortunate enough to have even that. This will give you some time to face the unhappy event you have lived through and will allow you to take the right decision for future.

Fear and insecurity are the other outcome of discontented state of mind. Fundamentally, we do not want to lose or part with things we already have and we are overcome by the feeling of fear. If we have a contented disposition, we will have the stillness and peace of mind to observe this basic fact that all is changing at every moment and this is how Patañjali has defined time. The change from one fraction of a second to the other is time (Part IV, Sūtra 33). Nothing stays the same forever. It is the time that makes the mighty tree from a seedling and a handsome young man or a beautiful woman from a little baby. Changes are normal in life and we learn to be contented despite them. It is not possible that only those changes, which are beneficial for you, will happen. This is the basic fact of existence we must learn to accept. It is not possible that there is no autumn, no death, no hair fall and no wrinkles. If this were to happen, then the time will come to a stop and there also will not be new babies, new leaves and flowers and so on. Therefore, learn to accept time as fundamental to existence and be cheerful and happy and not fearful and unhappy. So many human babies are born and so many people die everyday. When we lose someone who is very dear to us, the world seems to crumble down for us. But that is a very subjective aspect of the reality we are facing at that time. We ourselves notice that the world goes on as usual and even in our own life, the activities continue. We have to console ourselves in one way or the other and reach a level of contentment so that we can continue our life. The idea of this discussion is that you should make an effort to assimilate the fundamental wisdom of life so that you can save yourself from negative emotions like fear and insecurity that cause numerous disorders of all kinds.

All that which hinders development is *tamasic* in nature. The above-described emotions such as anger, envy, jealousy, competition, fear, insecurity and so on are *tamasic.* These thoughts hinder creativity and development in one way or the other. Modern life is dominated by *rajas* and there is no time left for sattvic values. When we make an effort to achieve a mental state of *santoṣa,* we get rid of the by-products of *asantoṣa* which are *tamasic.* In their absence, we become more tolerant, patient, courageous and generous. We feel at peace with ourselves and even the *rajas* activities are done with equilibrium, harmony and wisdom. Through our own experience, we realise that our efficiency enhances and this inspires us to seek more inner peace and stillness. The decisions we take at a *sattvic* level are always wiser than the ones we take in rage or anguish. The reason for this is that in the *sattvic* state, our mind is enlightened with the light of the soul and we are at a higher level of intellect. In very simple terms and language, we may say that brain works better that way. It is not only the higher level of intellect, but also the intuitive power develops with *sattva.* As is clear throughout

Patañjali's book, with the stillness of mind comes spiritual lucidity and one becomes capable of knowing the past and the present, and the hidden and the distant and so on. The above ideas are presented in a diagrammatic form in Figure 26.

Sattva in daily life

I have already given an exercise for the purification of the mind in Programme one. In the programme below, I will give some suggestions to bring *sattva* in your daily routine. These thoughts should be put in practice and should be a part of your life. Going to gurus, attending meditation sessions few hours a week is not sufficient to attain inner peace. You need to work on yourself persistently and make a constant effort to make yourself strong and stable person and to develop your higher faculties. In the tradition of yoga, it is said that a guru is there to show you the right path by teaching some techniques and helping you to remove some obstacles. The success lies in following that spiritual path with determination and perseverance to reach the desired destination. In the following programme, I give some very simple, almost non-time consuming suggestions that you can gradually incorporate in your daily routine.

Programme number three

Try to include the following points in your day's programme in such a way that they ultimately become your way of life. Take them one by one and try each for a week and then add the next to it.

An eight-fold programme for initiating *sattva*

1. Upon getting up in the morning, turn towards east and say few words of thankfulness to the Sun for giving you another day of life. Seek his blessings so that all your senses work until the end of your life and you may lead a long and fulfilled life.
2. Do all your morning activities by paying full attention to them, observe your excretions so that you can do your daily diagnosis of health as I have described elsewhere.[8]

---

[8] Refer to my book, *Āyurveda, A Way of Life,* Chapter 3.

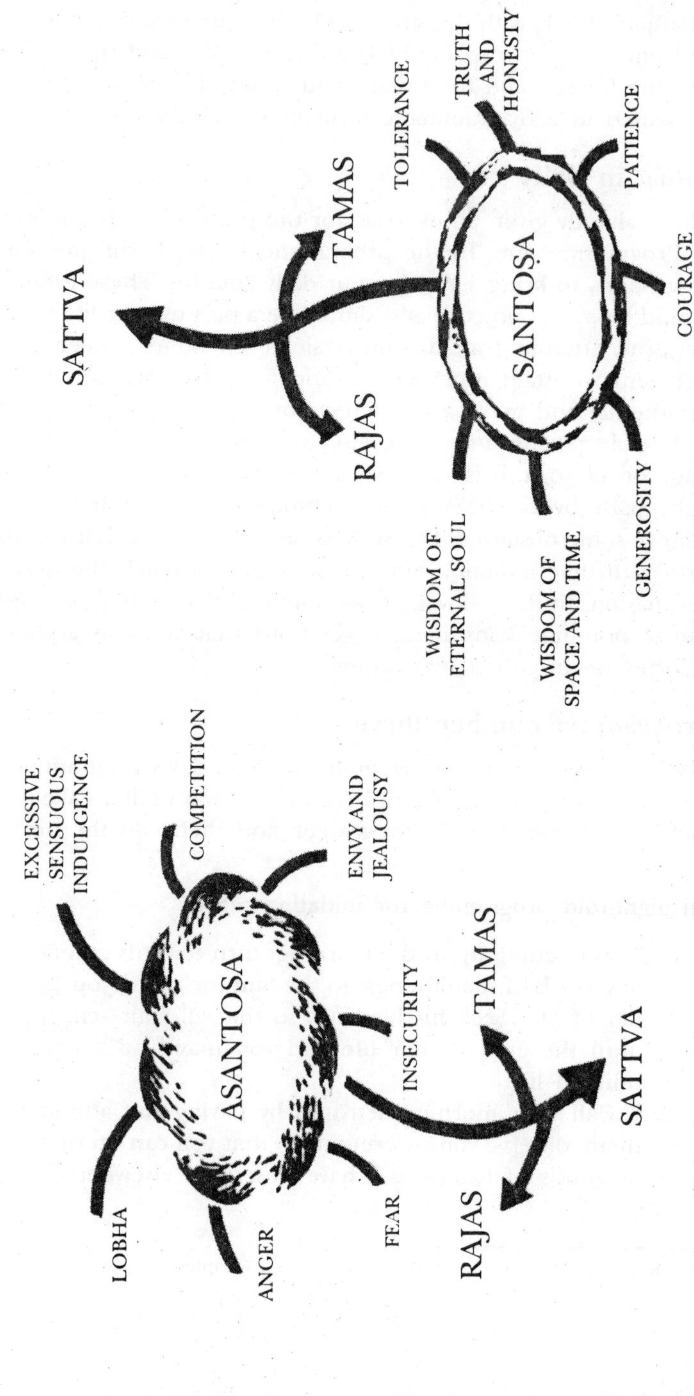

Figure 26. Suppression and rise of *sattva* with *asantoṣa* and *santoṣa* respectively.

3. Pay attention when you take a shower or a bath. Make a wish that along with the outer dirt from your body, the inner dirt may also part and may your mind be purified and you achieve inner peace and harmony. In case you have pain, malfunction or any other trouble in any part of your body, concentrate on the flowing water and make a wish that may the flowing water take this disorder away with it. May this disorder be thrown in the drain like the other dirt from your body.
4. Before eating each meal, take some deep breaths and say the prayers of gratefulness in one way or the other.
5. Before starting your day and going out of the house or starting your car each time, always take some deep breaths, touch something holy or a pure piece of silver or a crystal etc. Never lose your attention while driving and always take few deep breaths every now and then. Send the *prāṇa* energy to your head.
6. Do similar kind of breathing breaks throughout the day and send *prāṇa* energy to the part of your body that you may feel is fatigued. It is the matter of two three breaths every one or two hours and thus, it does not require any extra time.
7. Whenever you have an emotional outburst, do not lose contact with yourself. That means—observe yourself doing that activity. Your whole being should not get involved in that, you should be able to observe yourself getting angry, getting jealous, in a state of self-pity and so on. That way, you will be able to keep some control over yourself.
8. Before going to bed, bring yourself in harmony with night's energy and wish for a profound *rajas*- and *tamas*-free sleep. A state of sleep in which the inner stillness prevails and which is achieved after *prāṇāyāma* and while doing *japa* is called *yoganidrā*. With *yoganidrā*, one can get more rest only with few hours of sleep.

This is my simple, eight-fold programme to initiate you into a *sattvic* way of life. We will be discussing some of these aspects in more detail in the following Chapters.

CHAPTER 3

Āsanas and *Prāṇāyāma*

(The Yogic Postures and Breathing Exercises)

In Part II, Sūtras 46 and 47, Patañjali has described an *āsana* or yogic posture as follows:

> **'An *āsana* is that which is steady and pleasant. By effortlessness and by continuous intentness of mind, *āsana* becomes steady and pleasant.'**

To put it in very simple words, I would say an *āsana* is a particular body posture that is effortless, is stable, can be maintained for a while and is accompanied by a continuous intentness of mind. To achieve success in making an *āsana,* we also require to co-ordinate the breathing with any specific posture we are making.

According to Patañjali, after one has acquired mastery on yogic postures, a regulated inhalation and exhalation is practised and this is called *prāṇāyāma* (Part II, Sūtra 49).

With both, *āsanas* and *prāṇāyāma,* body and mind are strengthened, you feel at peace with yourself and are able to attain harmony with the cosmic energy. With a constant effort and practice, you are able to attain self-control, ability to break the chain of thoughts in mind and to get a thought-free mental state. Let us see in detail how these phenomena work to achieve a specific purpose.

The *āsanas* described in this book need flexibility of the body and an initial training in simpler *āsanas* as well as the very basic requisites for making an *āsana.* For this purpose, you may consult my book, *Yoga for Integral Health.* But in any case, for learning yogic practices, you need a teacher who can correct you and teach the techniques of achieving success in various *āsanas* and other practices. Sometimes, it can be dangerous to learn completely on your own exclusively with the help of books. We provide an extensive training in Āyurvedic yoga in our Āyurvedic courses in the Himalayan Centre. However, we do not take yoga as an exclusive theme because for health purposes, both are interdependent and should be adopted as a way of life. It is evident from Patañjali's eight-fold yoga that cleaning practices, restraint and self-discipline are essential before one learns *āsanas* and breathing practices. Besides, when someone has problems in making a particular *āsana*, for example, some pain and so on, then we need to apply the Āyurvedic principles to get rid of this obstruction. I do not mean to teach yogic practices to reduce weight which you have put on due to over-eating. The person concerned will have to learn to control first his/her sensuous desire and greed to over-eat. Then only the other methods of yoga should be applied to reduce weight.

Another prerequisite for the yogic practices is the purification of the body which has been the theme of last chapter. Like Āyurveda, yoga provides many purification practices and in fact in my last Āyurveda book, I have incorporated yogic purification practices in Āyurvedic *pañcakarma* practices. With dirt accumulated in the intestines, dirty tongue, stomach or the passages of the nose blocked, it is not possible to achieve success in *āsanas* or *prāṇāyāma*.

My purpose here is to teach you the essence of *āsanas* and *prāṇāyāma* so that you learn the 'soul' of Patañjali's yoga in practice. You can develop the ability to use the yogic practices to strengthen your body and mind, enhance the quality of life and prolong it, develop the ability to prevent ailments and heal and cure disorders.

Concept of an *āsana*

Before you learn to make yogic postures or *āsanas*, you should understand their scientific basis. By attempting to make an *āsana* without understanding its profound sense, you may not be able to get its real benefit and there is a fear of mechanically doing it merely as a physical exercise. Then, its purpose is defeated.

In our day to day life, we are used to our mind commanding our body. In Chapter 1 of this Section, exercises involving the legs are described. We see that the mind commands the leg to be lifted gradually in a steady manner. By repeating these movements again and again, we also slow down our thoughts. Gradually, mind develops the capability of commanding its own extensions in a very controlled manner. With repeated practice, it also develops a capacity to control the activities of the senses, which are also its extensions. The movements are an effort to reach the posture or *āsana*. Staying in a posture gives us training of stillness of mind. By making persistent effort to make a posture steady and comfortable, we put our mental energy into bodily organs. On the other hand we train our mind with our bodily organs. For example, we try each time to bring our leg a little higher which involves our mental persistence as well as physical persistence on the part of the leg. This physical persistence trains and strengthens our mind. At the scientific level, the central nervous system is capable of commanding the peripheral nervous system but I presume that the peripheral nervous system has also the capacity to influence the central nervous system. This is how gradually the communication between body and mind develops. The capability of body to communicate with the mind is very beneficial for us for preventing ailments. When we live in a mechanised manner, all actions take place under the command of the mind and under the precepts of the so-called rationality we have developed. Our rationality is based upon a pre-established theory that we take it as the ultimate truth. This theory is that the material reality is the only reality. When we live in a holistic manner, we explore and experience multiple dimensions of reality. This is how the ancient sages developed various methods to explore and use different dimensions of human energy. Thus, with *yogāsanas*, we make our body talk and register its condition on the mind. Mind and body stop imposing themselves on each other. They begin to be considerate to each other and co-ordinate with each other. By making different postures, we are able to 'feel' inner parts of our body and know immediately if there is any problem anywhere. For an appropriate *āsana*, a constant intentness of the mind is required and if the mind is disturbed, it acquires peace gradually with a constant bodily effort and its co-ordination with it.

To concentrate on an *āsana*, mind has to withdraw from the senses. In fact, to concentrate on anything, it has to withdraw from the external sensuous world and put all its intentness on one particular theme or whatever is the case. But while we are trying to make an *āsana*, in fact we are trying to control the movements of the body. I will give you a simpler example. I have developed some very simple exercises for my yoga classes so that people can be initiated into concentrating their mind on their body. These are very simple body movements. Put both your hand on the table or on your legs and clap them one by one in a rhythm of 1, 2, 3, 4. From 4, begin one again. A similar exercise can be done with your feet. You will see that you need full concentration of the mind to be able to continue this rhythm. The moment your thoughts are distracted, your rhythm will break. It is the effort to keep up this physical co-ordination which makes the mind concentrate.

We will take up some *yogāsanas* and I will explain step by step how an *āsana* is perfected. The idea here is to bring you to the realisation of what an *āsana* is. I have described many *āsanas* in all my books on Āyurveda and yoga. In the present context, the idea is to learn to reach perfection of an *āsana.* I will also describe some new *āsanas* for curing specific ailments.

Programme number four

Learning to make an āsana

In this programme, we will take the same example of the *āsanas* for legs, the *Uttānapāda āsanas* as in Programme number two. I will demonstrate that you will have to go through various stages and it requires will power and repetition to have success in making an *āsana.* Let us see all these in steps, in an analytical manner so that based on this knowledge, you are able to achieve success in whatever *āsana* you like.

Step 1: When you begin to lift your leg, your mind is involved in this effort and also you have to watch out that you are applying force at the right place and not bending your knee etc.

Step 2: Some of you may face difficulty and may not be able to lift the leg very high. There are others who may feel that this effort of lifting fatigues their abdominal muscles or the area of the pelvic joint. Some people can lift one leg more easily than the other, which speaks of imbalance in the two sides of the body. It is possible that some of you may not be able to co-ordinate breathing with the movements.

Step 3: Depending upon the extent of hurdles you have, you have to gradually get over them by making a little effort every day. Patañjali's yogic methods do not suggest the use of force with oneself; they teach us to achieve success with constant persistence. I also believe that with the use of force, some delicate persons may harm themselves and may end up getting muscular tension and pain.

Step 4: Let us imagine that you have reached a state when you can make all the movements smoothly and are also able to co-ordinate your breathing with the movements. You also feel at ease while your leg is up and do not feel exerted. At this stage, you are prepared to make this *āsana.* This state is generally taken to be an *āsana.* The actual *āsana* is to be able to stay with ease in the position with the leg upward while your thought process is fully concentrated on this action. For staying long, you do not have to hold your breath, the slow and short breathing will take place automatically. You should be able to stay effortlessly in this position. The body should be relaxed and free of tension. Always rest for a period of five to ten breaths after you have come back to the normal position from an *āsana.*

Benefits of an *āsana*

I hope that with the above description, you have well understood what an *āsana* is supposed to be. It is to attain the flexibility and ease in a particular position to the extent that you feel comfortable with it; you may not feel tense or breathless and are able to devote all your mental attention to this posture. Benefits of different *āsanas* are different but here I will describe in general what an *āsana* does at diverse levels.

1. Various *āsanas* help in smooth blood flow in the body and remove obstructions, if any, from the blood vessels. For example, when you stay with the leg or legs up for a while in a constant and stable manner, your blood is diverted towards the upper parts of your body with force. You feel the heat in your arms and head region. In diverse *āsanas,* the blood is thoroughly circulated in all parts of the body. Besides this, all the internal organs get appropriate stretching and revitalisation. If there is any slightest of problem in any part of the body, one is able to detect it. Taking the above example of the leg *āsanas,* if you have one leg weaker than the other, or shorter than the other, or some problem with the pelvic joint or related muscles, you are able to detect and take an appropriate treatment. Since your mind is also completely concentrated on the *āsana* you are making, it becomes capable of exploring the inside of your body. The *yogāsanas* have revitalising and rejuvenating effect on the body.
2. Mind-body closeness develops and you learn to divert the mental energy on various parts of your body. This training

is very essential for mental and spiritual therapy. This subject will be discussed later in the book.

3. The five fundamental elements; which make the material reality of our cosmos as well as of our body, are symbolically distributed in the body. Earth is between feet and knees, water is between knees and anus, fire is between anus and plexus, air is between plexus and eyebrows and ether is between eyebrows and top of the head. These elements are distributed in the order of their weight (see Table 2). By making diverse positions, we do the energy exchange between all the five elements in different parts of our body. For example, with the legs up, we send the energy of the earth and water into rest of our body. The earth represents our roots and our stability. When in another *āsana*, we are standing and touching our feet with our hands, we are bringing the energy of the lighter elements to the earth. Diverse *yogāsanas* help to re-establish humoral balance as these three vital forces are made of the five fundamental elements. I will talk of this again in the context of diverse *āsanas* as well as in healing various ailments.

By going into such analytical details, I wish to bring across to you that if you will not learn *yogāsanas* or other yogic practices in an appropriate manner, their benefits for health will be only to a limited extend. My principal purpose to make this theme of Āyurvedic yoga and write this part of the book is to put across as a comprehensible subject that can be understood and used in everyday life for preventing and healing ailments and for curing various disorders.

Let us take up the next *āsana* now!

Programme number five

Uttānapṛṣṭhavaṃśa āsanas to strengthen the digestive fire (agni) and the backbone

1. Try this *āsana* only after you have attained mastery over *uttānapāda āsana* as it also involves lifting up of both the legs along with upper part of the body (Figure 27). Your body weight is balanced on your lower half of the back and your forearm. To make this *āsana*, lie down on your back with arms stretched out and feet joined together. Gradually

lift your head as well as both your legs with both the feet joined together. Take the support of your elbows as shown in the figure.

2. Lie down on your back with your arms stretched upwards and your feet joined together. Lift upwards both your arms and legs simultaneously. Head and the back will lift slightly in this process (Figure 28).
3. Lie down on your back with your hands under your head and the fingers clasped together. Your feet should be joined together, as was the case in the above two exercises. Lift up your back and head as if you are getting up from the supine position (Figure 29). Your body weight in this case will be on the lower part of the back.

Practice all these three *āsanas* until you have mastery over them according to the description given in the previous programme. These three *āsanas* are for curing digestive problems and for revitalising the digestive fire (agni). They strengthen the backbone and back muscles. You will see that each of them specifically acts on different parts of the back in different manners.

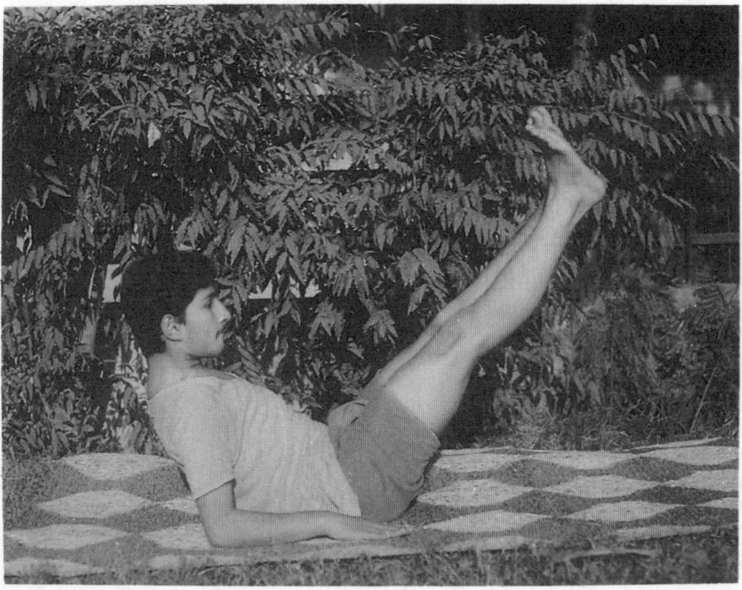

Figure 27. *Uttānapṛṣṭhavaṃśa āsana* 1.

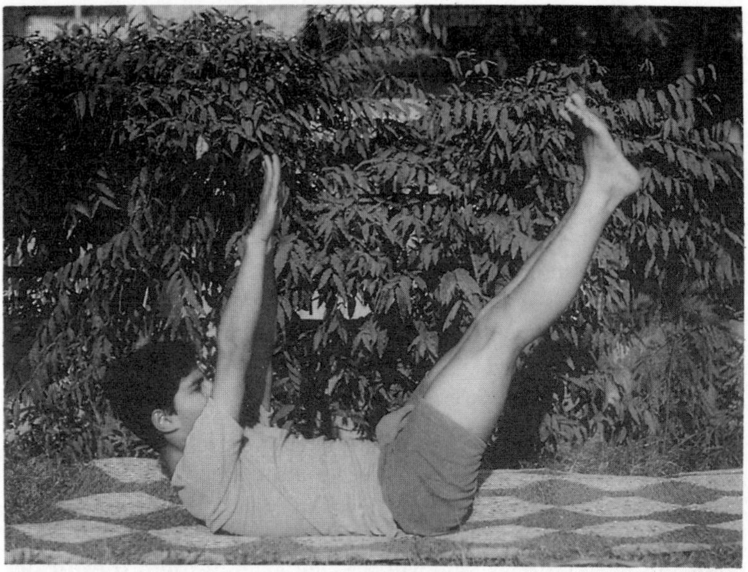

Figure 28. *Uttānapṛṣṭhavaṃśa āsana* 2.

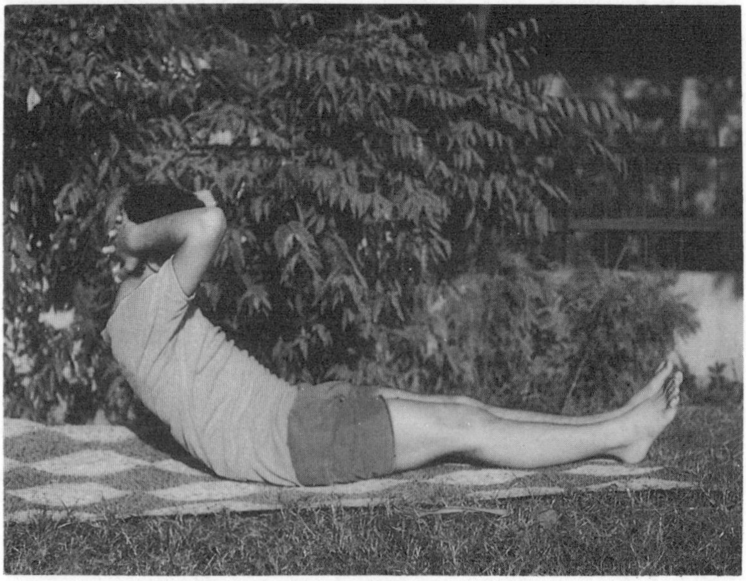

Figure 29. *Uttānapṛṣṭhavaṃśa āsana* 3.

Note: If you have back or neck pains or any other pain related to the backbone, you should not do these āsanas. You should first cure your problems with the six backbone āsanas I have described previously in my book, Sixteen Minutes to a Better 9-to-5.

Programme number six

Āsanas to revitalise the digestive fire

Like in the above *āsanas,* this series of *āsanas* also rejuvenate the digestive fire- that means the power to digest, digestive juices, the capacity to assimilate and so on. For details of the digestive fire or agni, you may consult my book, *Āyurveda, a Way of Life,* Chapter 2.

1. The first *āsana* of this series is very simple and most of you may already know about it, as it is a very popular *āsana.* It is called *Bhujaṅgāsana* or the cobra or serpent *āsana* and involves lifting up your head and chest while you lie down on your stomach. Lie down on your stomach and let your chin rest on the floor. Put your hands nearly at the level of your chest and your arms will bend in this process. Now lift your head and chest gradually while inhaling. Bend as far back as you comfortably can and straighten your arms (Figure 30). Initially stay only for few seconds in this posture and your breath is held inside during this time. Bring your

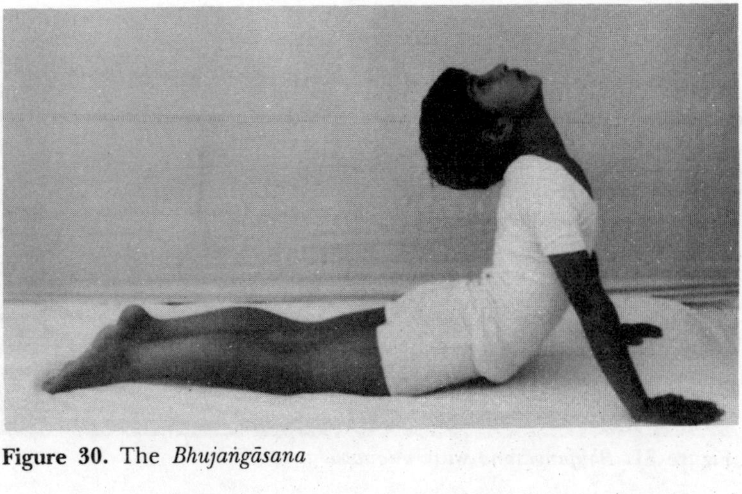

Figure 30. The *Bhujaṅgāsana*

head and chest downwards gradually while you exhale.
As in the other *āsana*, with persistent practice, you may perfect it. When you prolong the duration of this *āsana*, you will have a very superficial and slow breathing. Some of the air is trapped in the deeper parts of the lungs while you are in this position.
Besides curing digestive problems and revitalising the body fire, this āsana is indispensable for curing chronic cough and asthma.

2. The second *āsana* of this series involves two of the bodily skills you have learnt in two different *āsanas* previously. Lie down on your stomach as described above. Lift up your head and chest and one of your legs simultaneously. In this *āsana*, your arms are not straightened like in the previous one (Figure 31). By keeping a gap of few breaths, repeat the *āsana* with the other leg. As said previously, enhance the duration of the *āsana* by a regular practice.
This *āsana* also energises your shoulders, arms and legs.
3. In this *āsana*, you make your body like a bow and this *āsana* is called *Dhanurāsana*. Lie down on your stomach. Bend your legs from the knees and bring your ankles as close to your hips as possible. Stretch back your arms and hold your ankles with your hands. Tighten the grip and lift up your body by applying force from the hands and arms (Figure 32). As in the other above-described *āsanas*, breathing

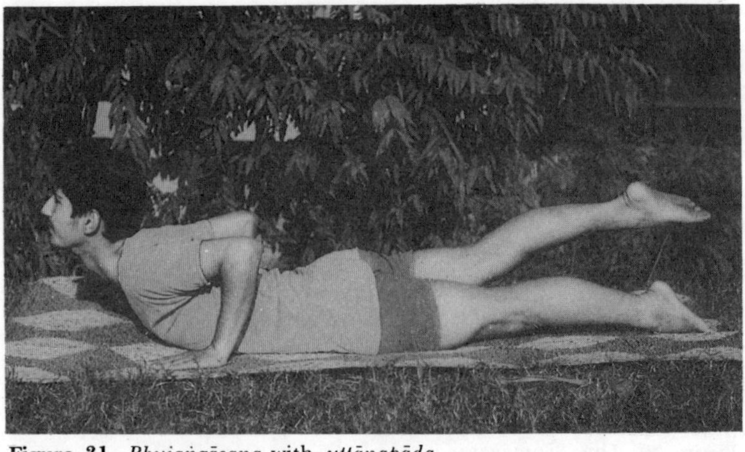

Figure 31. *Bhujaṅgāsana* with *uttānapāda*.

is superficial and slow when you stay longer in this *āsana*. I do not want to confuse you by talking too much about breathing in this *āsanas* as the respiration process automatically regulates according to the shape the body acquires and the possibility of inhalation available in the given circumstances. However, you should never forget to realise your limitation and never go beyond your capacity in any case. Success should come with gradual practice.

4. This *āsana* is called *khagāsana* or bird posture and is a further development of number 3. While your body is in the shape of a bow, rock yourself forward and backward with the part that is touching the ground (see arrows on Figure 32).

In the above two *āsanas*, the whole body is involved and they energise all the internal organs of the body, muscles and joints.

Programme number seven

Some whole-body āsanas

For the benefit of the body in totality, I will describe below four *āsanas*, which involve whole of your body. Increase gradually the

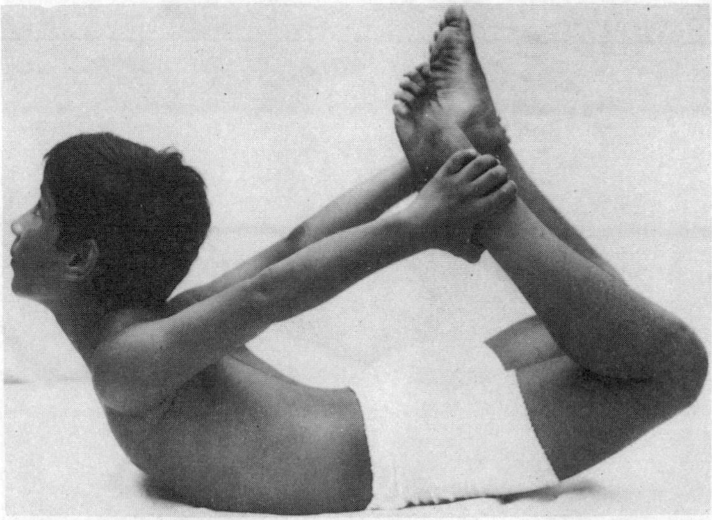

Figure 32. *Dhanurāsana.*

duration to stay in these *āsanas* and keep the concentration of the mind while in the posture. Hinder the flow of thoughts and only the form of the body in that posture should be in your mind.

1. This *āsana* is called *Halāsana* or plough *āsana*, as your body will make a shape resembling a plough. Lie on your back with feet together and arms slightly apart from the body. When you are completely relaxed, start raising both your legs as you have learnt in the leg *āsanas*. For making this *āsana*, raise your legs further and touch the ground beyond your head (Figure 33). Do not make your arms or hands tense. Repeat until you achieve perfection and feel comfortable.
2. This *āsana* is in fact another version of the plough *āsana*. The only difference is that in this you stretch your arms upwards and then touch your hands with your feet (Figure 34).
3. This *āsana* is called the *Sarvāṅgāsana* or the whole-body *āsana*. Some compare it to the flame of a candle. Lie down in the same position as in number 1 and start lifting up

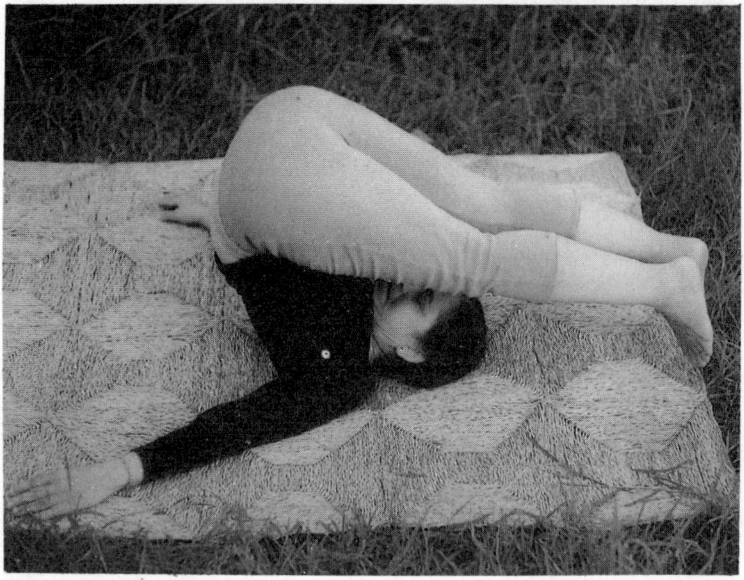

Figure 33. *Halāsana* 1.

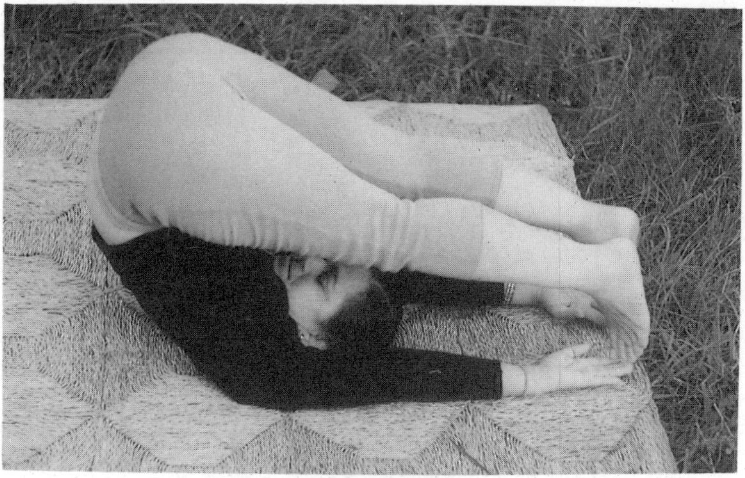

Figure 34. *Halāsana* 2.

your legs. When your legs are at a right angle to your body, give a slight pause and then bring them towards your head. Your waist will be raised in this process. Put both your hands on your waist to provide a support and stretch whole of your body upwards. Your body should be in a straight line and your body weight is supported by your neck and shoulders (Figure 35). Normally, your chin will press against your chest. To come to the normal position from this *āsana*, first bend your legs towards your head, remove the support of your hands and let your back gradually descend on the ground. Make an effort to achieve perfection in this posture.

4. This *āsana* is called *Uṣṭrāsana* or camel posture. You make your whole body circular in it. Sit on your knees while your legs are bent backwards. In fact, it is like half standing on your knees. Stretch your arms backwards and also bend your body backwards and touch your feet with your hands as shown in Figure 36.

After each of these *āsanas*, you should relax and lie down in *śavāsana* or the dead body posture. This posture is made by lying down on your back in a completely relaxed manner and letting yourself loose to such an extent as if you were a dead body. Are you afraid? It is an extremely relaxing posture and refreshes you

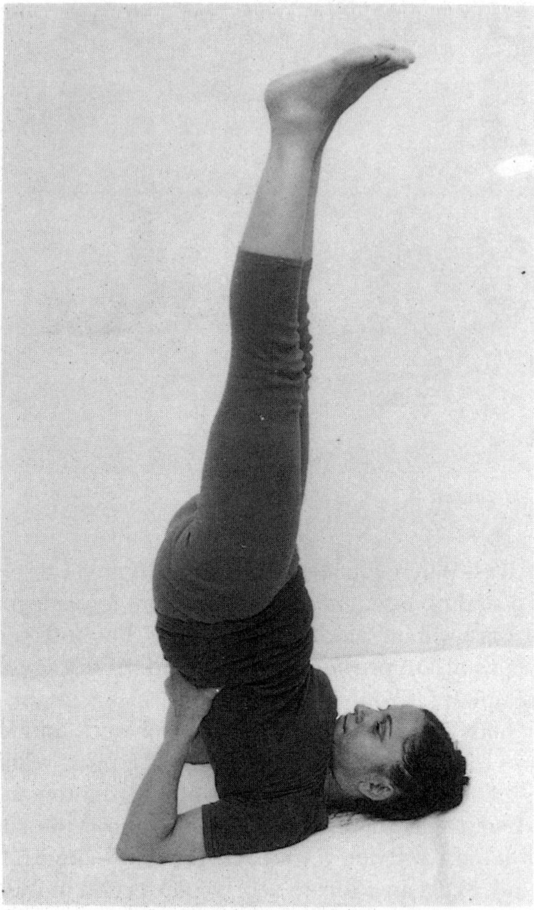

Figure 35. *Sarvāṅgāsana.*

for the next posture. For details of making this posture, you may consult my book *Yoga for Integral Health.*

Programme number eight

The two standing āsanas

I am mentioning these *āsanas* particularly for those situations when you have no place to practice your *āsanas,* but you can at least revitalise your body upon getting up in the morning. In such

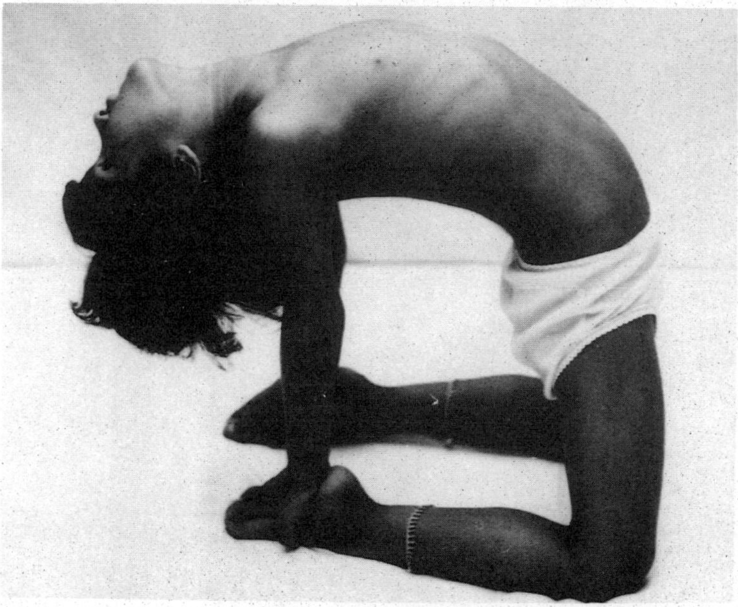

Figure 36. *Uṣṭrāsana.*

situations like travelling or having little time because of being busy and so on, you may at least do the stretching exercises described earlier in Programme number 1 along with these two *āsanas.*

1. Stand straight with feet slightly apart from each other. Put your palms on the lower part of your back and bend as much backward as you can (Figure 37). Return gradually in the standing posture.
2. In this posture, the movement of the body is in the reverse direction of the above. While you are standing straight, put both your arms upwards so that they are parallel to each other. Bend forwards to touch your feet with your hands (Figure 38). Your knees should not bend in this *āsana.* If your body is flexible, you are able to touch your knees with your head.

What is *prāṇāyāma*?

The literal meaning of *prāṇāyāma* is to develop control over one's *prāṇa. Prāṇa* means life itself or consciousness. The cause of

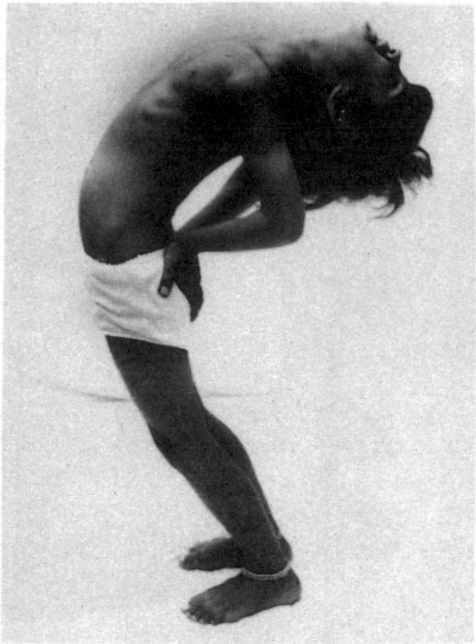

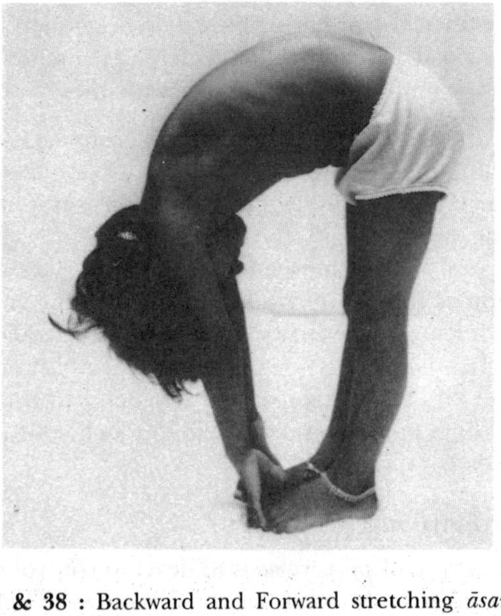

Figures 37 & 38 : Backward and Forward stretching *āsana*.

consciousness is soul in the body but the factor that holds body and soul together and is responsible for a continuous vivacity is *prāṇa*. When *prāṇa* stops, the body and soul separate and death occurs. *Prāṇa* or a continuous cosmic energy comes to us through our breathing process. Thus, breathing is not simply a mechanical phenomenon that gives fuel in the form of oxygen for making the body-machine work as is thought by those who compare living body to a machine. The phenomenon of breathing is our link with the cosmos and in the form of air we inhale cosmic energy and not merely the required oxygen. The five fundamental elements and five subtle elements are a part of this energy with which we perform five kinds of actions through our five sense organs (see Table 2 for the details of twentyfive elements of *Sāṃkhya*). Thus, when we learn to control the *prāṇa* energy, we can develop the ability to divert it in different directions for beneficial purpose. Yoga has very sophisticated techniques of teaching us to harness this energy. But the importance of this energy is well known also in many other cultures of the world and marshal arts of Asia. During many natural processes of the body and its various activities like excretion, sexuality, expression of anger or other emotions, our breathing acquires various forms. We all know how the breathing alters during sexuality and the sensuous pleasure is related to the breathing phenomena. I have discussed this theme in details in my book- *The Kāmasūtra for Women.*

Let me explain more explicitly what I mean when I say that the air we inhale has cosmic energy and we need all of it with its specific constituents and not just oxygen as is believed in modern biology and medicine. The definition of being alive may also differ in modern and holistic medicine. From the holistic point of view, being alive is being conscious and having the discriminative power or intellect (*buddhi*). For example, persons in coma or when kept alive with artificial breathing and nourishing are alive only in a limited biological sense. Anyhow, coming back to the theme of *prāṇa*, it is important to know that it is not the exclusive air we are taking inside us each time we breathe. That air we inhale exists in certain space. In fact, space or ether is one element, which is a prerequisite to any existence. All what exists cannot be separated from ether. Thus, we inhale ether and ai both. The third element is fire, and we take it inside us in th form of heat of the atmosphere. Imagine yourself always breathing in the air that is kept at below zero or above 70°C. Even the thought of it is unpleasant. Thus, the equilibrium of the fire element in the air we inhale is essential. The fourth fundamental element is water and we all know that the inhalation of the absolutely dry air will cause haemorrhage in our nasal passage and may also lead to other severe complications. The water element is essential and is always there in the air we inhale.

A large part of the air is made of nitrogen, which makes the substantial part of our body in the form of proteins. There are many other elements of earth (carbon, silicon, calcium, phosphorus etc.) in the air. Since we have all the fundamental elements in the atmosphere from which we breathe in, the related subtle elements are also obviously taken in. The vital quality of the air changes with time of the day, weather, climate etc. and that effects directly our lives. We must remember that the intake of vital air is a phenomenon, which is linked with our whole life— it is life itself and that is why the sages called it *prāṇa.*

Besides all that I have described above, we have also all kinds of gases, many kinds of waves like magnetic, electronic and so on, fungus, algae or spores of other plants, bacteria, virus, pollen and infinite number of other substances in the air. By regulating our breath and controlling its journey into our being, we, therefore, control our cosmic interaction with our mental and physical processes and learn to influence them with the cosmic energy. We can use the cosmic energy for healing as well as to control our mental state.

Patañjali says that a regular inhalation and exhalation with intervals is *prāṇāyāma* and should be practised only after attaining mastery over the *āsanas.* He further tells us three parts of *prāṇāyāma*—the inhalation, exhalation and the absence of these two. The later sages termed these three as *recaka, pūraka* and *kumbhaka* respectively and this is the popular terminology that is used until today. *Kumbhaka* or the absence of inhalation and exhalation has two aspects- one is to hold the air inside and the other is to hold the lungs without air. Further, Patañjali adds that after a long time of practice, the fourth stage of *prāṇāyāma* is achieved where there is very little difference between the movement and the stillness of the breath. That means that the inhalation and exhalation are reduced to such a degree that the restraint of breath is spontaneously achieved. When this is achieved, the cover of darkness from around the source of light i.e. soul, is removed. The cover of darkness is not to recognise the eternal energy, the cause of consciousness as our real self and instead identify oneself with the destructible, non-eternal body. (Part II, Sūtras 49-52).

In the present context of Āyurvedic yoga, our aim is slightly different than that of Patañjali's yogī who seeks salvation from this world. However, the initial path in both the cases is the same, which is to achieve good health, harmony and a sense of well-being. *Prāṇāyāma* forms the basis of Āyurvedic spiritual healing and the practices you will learn will be used for diagnostic and healing purposes and this theme will be treated later in this book.

Prāṇic energy and its assimilation

I have already stated that respiration is not merely a simple physiological phenomenon but the vital force that keeps the body and soul together and keeps us alive. We experience one time or the other in our lives how fragile and precious this connection of *prāṇa* is. For example if your throat gets choked accidentally with food or water and for a moment you are unable to breathe, the life line seems very fragile. It gives sometimes a very brief experience of what death would be like. People suffering from chronic cough or asthma may also have this experience from time to time. There may be other similar incidents in one's life when one realises the extent of fragility with which life is connected to the body.

Before learning the *prāṇāyāma* techniques, you should learn to assimilate the *prāṇa* energy in you each moment. Try to observe your breathing very carefully. You will begin to realise how it alters during different emotional situations and during different activities. For example, if you are watching a movie or theatre with a fearful scene or any other situation with which you feel extremely involved, your breath will slow down and also stop for a moment at a decisive event. Observe this for first few days and follow your breath with your thoughts.

Try and get into the habit of breathing regularly and deeply. Also when you have an emotional situation or an event which completely engrosses you. Break your thoughts to assure that you are breathing deeply and in a rhythmical manner. This way, you will be able to assimilate more cosmic energy. To make you comprehend better, I will give you an example from food. In Āyurveda, it is not only the quality or quantity of food that is discussed but also the manner it should be consumed. If you eat quickly while standing or walking or while under stress, this food will not do you any good. Your body may not get the full worth of food and it may not be assimilated properly. If you continue to do so over the years, you may end up getting digestive problems. On the other hand, the same food taken in a good atmosphere, with proper decor and with a peaceful mental state after having taken few deep breaths and so on, will assimilate properly and will provide you energy and radiance. Similarly, from the abundance cosmic energy, if you do not inhale and exhale properly and with appropriate pauses, you may get a pale look, may get prone to throat or other respiratory tract infection and get easily fatigued. Therefore, practice and repeatedly check yourself to breathe in an appropriate yogic manner.

Variations in *prāṇic* energy

According to Āyurveda, different geographical locations, climatic conditions, our age and different times of the day have different effect on us in terms of the three humours. Therefore, we should live according to time and space besides living with our fundamental nature (*Prakṛti*). Similarly, the *prāṇic* energy varies in different times of the day, different climatic and geographical conditions. Its quality also depends upon the vegetation of the particular regions and so on. The breathing pattern of an individual also varies in sleep and wakeful states, according to the humidity level, heat, height of the place and so on. For a holistic physician, amongst other things, there is also importance of climate and change of place for cure and therapy. Besides the effect of these factors on the three humours, the importance is also of the change in the *prāṇic* energy. In simple terms, we assimilate weather, climate etc. through our intake of *prāṇa*. When we talk about the effect of all these factors on our health and mind, it is at two different levels, physiological and subtle, which of course are interconnected and interdependent. Here I do not mean in the sense of polluted or non-polluted atmosphere; I am assuming the non-polluted atmosphere with natural variations. The polluted atmosphere causes, what I call, the vitiation of the *prāṇa* energy and I will take up this theme later.

I will give some concrete examples to make you understand the variations in *prāṇic* energy and its effect on us. In summer in Europe or during monsoons in India, after few hot days, sometimes clouds appear but they do not rain. The sky stays cloudy for one or two days. I will not go into the measurable details like the air pressure a barometer, as my idea is to make you experience nature. Thus, the clouds are there but there is no rain and the air is still. You will feel a kind of tension in the atmosphere. You will feel this tension in your mind and body also. For example, you may get constipation to some degree depending upon your Āyurvedic nature. Your menstruation may be delayed. You may find yourself tense and this may display itself in your interaction with other persons for that brief period of time. Release and outflow of thoughts, emotions, actions and biological processes may get delayed. Once there is rain, you experience a feeling of relief in every respect. Essentially, the tension or the state of the atmosphere affects us in the form of *prāṇic* energy. We are connected to the cosmos with *prāṇa* as I have said already and through this we are directly linked to the atmospheric state. The state of *prāṇic* energy affects all what is there in the phenomenal world and that also includes the vegetation, water and other things we consume. Therefore the variation in *prāṇic* energy invades all and our being in every respect.

Generally, women have pre-menstrual tension in one way or the other. This is their inner atmosphere that is affecting the state of their body and mind. In the above example, it is the outer atmosphere, which affects our body and mind. Similarly, other changes in the entire cosmos affect us through *prāṇic* energy. It also includes different seasons, constellation of the planets, stars, day of the moon and so on. The night's *prāṇic* energy is quiet, inactive and *tamasic.* The early morning atmosphere is *sattvic* as the atmosphere is still not filled with sounds, noises and physical movements and mental unrest of people. *Prāṇic* energy in the mountains or forest is different than in and around the big cities where it is normally vitiated.

In 1991, there was a big earthquake here in Uttarkashi in the Himalayan Mountains where our Himalayan centre is and where I am writing this part of the book. The earthquake was in the night at around 2 o'clock. It is amazing that many people had woken up just before the earthquake. I made a thorough study of this and it turned out that in many incidents, it was children who asked for either water or for relieving themselves or they complained of some pain somewhere. My theory is that the pre-earthquake tension in the atmosphere was built and people perceived it through *prāṇic* energy.

Prāṇa Vikṛti

Prāṇa from the atmosphere goes in us every moment and provides us with abundance of energy— that is what I have said above. But sometimes, we human beings create an imbalance in the space around us by adding to it various pollutants, noise, smoke and many other filthy substances which disturb the balance of the cosmic energy in it. The sun and the moon acquire coppery appearance and the energy of the cosmic bodies does not reach our atmosphere properly. This is a state of *vikṛti* of *prāṇa* in the atmosphere. In other words, we may say that in such situations, as is the case in the most big cities in the world, many ailments may be caused because of the *prāṇa vikṛti* (vitiation) in the atmosphere. This gives rise to many disorders and untimely death. The cosmic energy does not reach in appropriate proportion and quantity at such places and due to that the vegetation cannot flourish properly. When we eat the food grown in these conditions, it is unable to supply us with required *prāṇa* energy and consequently despite the full measurable value of these nutrients, people feel fatigued and acquire a pale look without any radiance. This lack of life's energy further leads to behavioural changes in people and ultimately there is degeneration of health as well as intellect.

The *prāṇa* energy interacts with the green trees; it causes sounds of rustling of leaves, comes in contact with butterflies, birds and their chirping, the sounds of the rivers, water sources, fountains, rain, clouds and so on. But when we live in air-conditioned rooms and other closed and noisy places, and the *prāṇa* energy we inhale comes in contact with the noise of the machines and the motor vehicles around us, it has certainly another effect on us. We must remember that we not only hear noise, we also inhale it along with of course the gases and other pollutants which we also smell. Similarly, visually, when we see around us only cement buildings, human beings in abundance and no greenery and birds, it is not only the sense of sight which consumes all this, we also inhale this hardness of the surroundings every moment of our existence.

Thus, for good health, we not only need balance of the three humours and the three qualities of mind but also a balance in our atmosphere from which we inhale the *prāṇa* energy all the time. For preventing the vitiation of *prāṇa*, a joint effort from all of us at the universal level is required. The atmosphere on our planet earth cannot be selectively saved or destroyed as with strong winds, water currents, sea waves and so on, the pollution travels from one place to another. The fertilisers and pesticides that are destroying us by slow poisoning are never limited to their place of origin. Similarly, other polluting products are taken all over the world by traders, like chemicals in food preservation, soaps, toothpastes, shampoos etc. Therefore, we need to form international bodies with devoted and dynamic people for this cause, which can function effectively to free the atmosphere from the vitiation of the *prāṇa* energy.

The *prāṇa* inside us

In the explanation of Sūtra 39, Part III, the fivefold action of the *prāṇa* inside the body has been described. These are as follows: 1) *prāṇa* is conducting the vital air through the mouth and nose up to the plexus; 2) *samāna* is conducting the vital air from plexus to the navel region; 3) *apāna* is conducting the vital air from navel region to the great toe; 4) *udāna* is conducting the vital air upwards to the head; 5) *vyāna* is conducting the vital air everywhere in the body.

Before you learn to direct *prāṇa* to specific levels of your body as described above, it is essential to learn the techniques which help to regulate, control and direct the *prāṇa* energy into the body. This is what *prāṇāyāma* is as has been stated in the beginning of this Chapter. I have already initiated you in observing your breath and inhaling it regularly. After having done that, in the following programme you will learn to direct it little more specifically with appropriate pauses. I have described these initial practices in several of my books earlier, but will repeat again briefly before you begin to learn about the *prāṇāyāma* practices of higher level.

Programme number nine

Initiation into prāṇāyāma

Step 1: In this step, simply learn to do the four steps of *prāṇāyāma* as Patañjali has described in Part II, Sūtra 49. Sit down cross-legged or in lotus posture. Make sure that your backbone is straight and your body is completely relaxed. Begin to inhale in a regular but gradual manner until nearly to your total capacity. Keep your entire concentration on the *prāṇa,* its rhythm and follow its journey inside you. At this stage, let yourself loose from the effort of inhalation and stay still while the *prāṇa* is inside you. Keep it in as long as you can and then exhale gradually with the same rhythm. Let your concentration not divert from your breath. When you have exhaled completely, stay without air a little and concentrate on your inner space. Repeat this whole process several times and gradually increase the timings of inhalation and exhalation as well as of holding with air and without it. The time of inhalation and exhalation should be the same and that of holding should be half of that. It does not mean that you should look at a watch, it is to give you the idea and the exactness of the technique.

Step 2: After the initial practice of Step 1, energise separately the left and right side of the body with *prāṇa.* These two sides represent *tamas* and *rajas* in the body respectively. They can also be compared to moon (left) and sun (right). This practice is done by closing one nostril and breathing exclusively with the other like described above for all the four parts of the *prāṇāyāma.* Pick up your right hand and close your right nostril with your thumb and inhale through your left nostril (Figure 39). Then hold the air inside by closing also your left nostril with your ring finger (Figure 40). Now lift your ring finger and exhale from the left side and replace the ring finger again to hold the lungs without air. Repeat the procedure six to ten times exclusively with left nostril. Make sure that your right nostril is kept closed properly. Later, repeat the same for the right nostril while you keep your left nostril closed.

Step 3: In this step, you inhale through the right nostril first while the left is closed with your thumb. Then close also the right nostril with your ring finger to hold the air inside. Let the air out through the left nostril by lifting the finger and continue to keep the

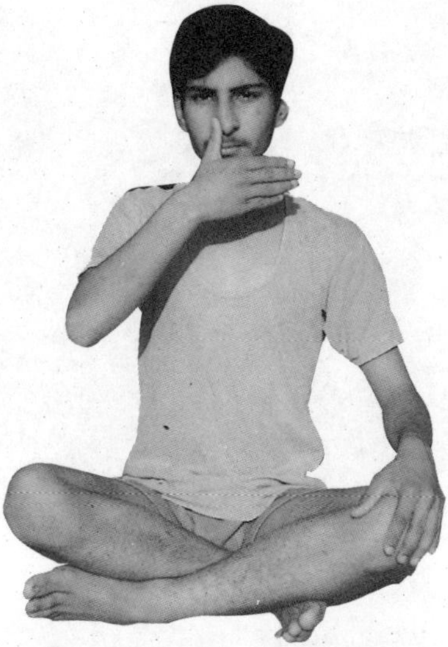

Figure 39. The initial practices of *prāṇāyāma.*

thumb on the right nostril. Close also the left nostril now to keep the lungs without air. Now the next time, inhale through the left nostril and continue the procedure. In other words, you inhale through one nostril and exhale through the other and for the next round, you inhale through the nostril through which you have previously exhaled. Repeat this also six to ten times.

Step 4: In this step, you do the inhalation through both the nostrils but close them with your thumb and ring finger when you have inhaled and when you are holding the lungs without air. This step will help you to prolong the timings of the four steps of *prāṇāyāma.*

Programme number ten

Practice of prāṇāyāma

Step 1: During the initiation, you were busy with the technical details of *prāṇāyāma.* With the repeated practice of the above steps, you succeed in prolonging the timings of all the four steps and are also able to concentrate. In this programme, you will learn to perform step 2 to 4 but without closing your nostrils. With practice, you will learn to breathe through one nostril but without

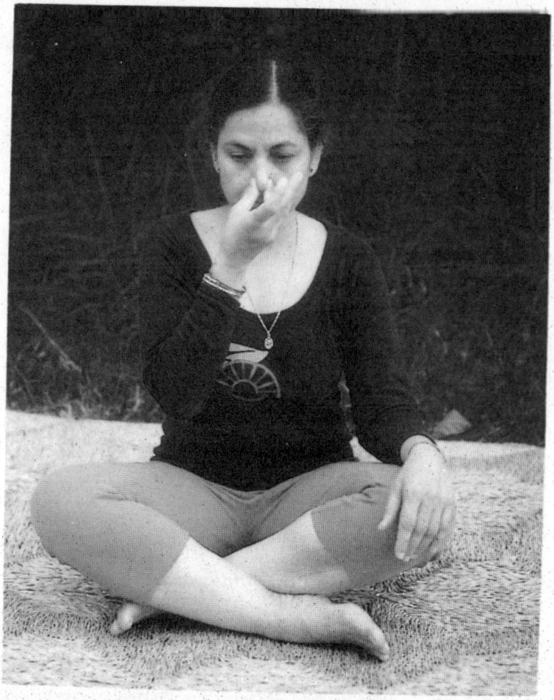

Figure 40. The initial practices of *prāṇāyāma.*

closing it and will also be able to hold air inside or hold the lungs without air without closing both your nostrils. This stage of *prāṇāyāma* is reached with constant practice, strong will and perseverance.

You need to immerse yourself completely in the process of the intake of *prāṇa* when you are trying to inhale or exhale through one nostril without closing the other.

Step 2: In this step, you have to learn to direct the *prāṇa* energy to a specific part of your body. Take the *prāṇa* in gradually and smoothly. Direct it to a specific part of the body. To begin with, guide the *prāṇa* to the plexus. Later, with practice, learn to direct the *prāṇa* to different parts of your body. If you are able to do it successfully, you will feel some heat or inner movement in that part of the body where you direct the *prāṇa*. Try a number of times, as you may not succeed immediately. Make an effort to direct *prāṇa* to different parts of your body like your arms, hands, fingers, feet etc. This way, you will learn to feel the *prāṇic* energy and its movement in different parts of your body and will be able to control it to the desired part on requirement. This requirement may be at two different levels. You may wish to rejuvenate some particular part like your cold hands and feet in winter or you may wish to evoke the *prāṇic* energy in a particular region of the body and use it for diagnosis or healing of ailments or making a protective covering around oneself. About this latter aspect, I will deal in details later in the book.

Programme number eleven

Advanced prāṇāyāma

It is only possible to learn this programme if you have attained mastery over the previous steps. In this programme, you will learn to perform certain activities with *prāṇa* which work at inner parts of the body as well as at the subtle energy level.

1. Stand straight with your legs slightly apart from each other. Bend forward and put your hands at your knees. Throw out your breath through the nasal passage with great force and while doing that pull inwards your lower part of the abdomen (Figure 41). Keep it as long as you can in this position.

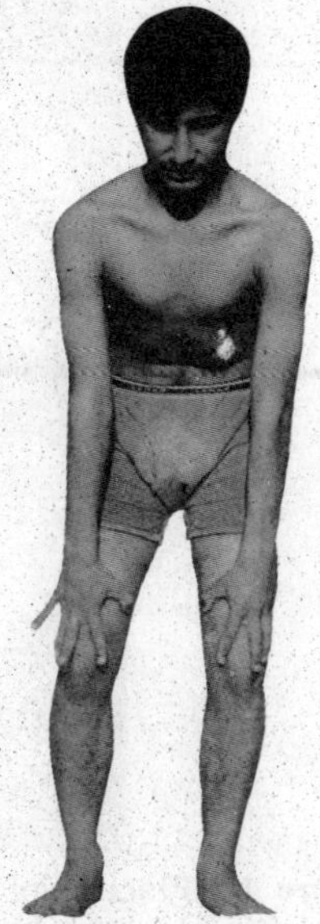

Figure 41. Practice of advanced *prāṇāyāma*.

In the beginning, do it only a few times and increase the duration and frequency gradually.

2. When you gain experience in doing the above practice, then in the same position, try to push out upper part of your abdomen in a similar way. The next step is to pull and push the lower and upper parts of the abdomen alternatively. These two practices are very useful for stomach but are difficult to learn. It is suggested that you take the help of a teacher to learn them.
3. In this practice, you inhale normally through the nasal passage but throw out the air with force through the mouth by making it like crow's beak with your lips while standing in the similar position as above (Figure 42).

   This practice is very beneficial for healing. It is used with a strong wish to throw out any disorder or ailment one is

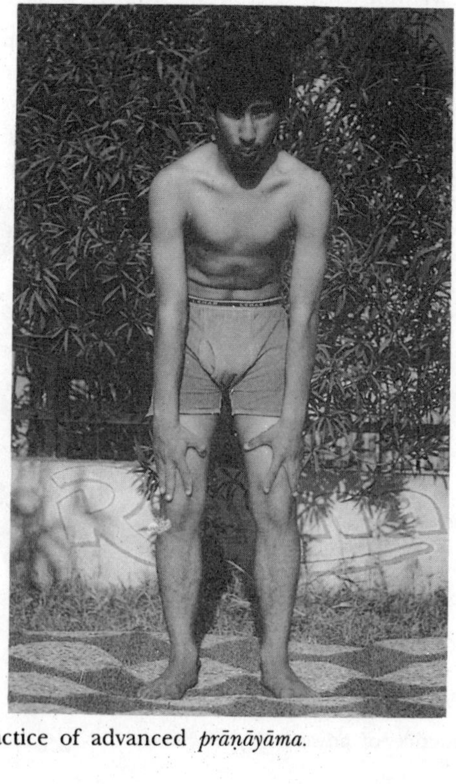

Figure 42. Practice of advanced *prāṇāyāma.*

suffering from. You concentrate on the ailing part and then draw upwards the ailment from it and throw it out with great force. There are some situations when you do such a gesture with reflex. For example, if a mosquito or other insect enters your mouth, you very strongly try to throw it out. You have to do movements of the air to bring it out as well as you curl your lips to apply the force. In this practice, you are throwing out also something that does not belong to your body, which is unpleasant and causing ill effects on your body. The strength and concentration of the mind should be applied along with the force of *prāṇa* to throw out the ailment along with the air. You need to repeat this process several times to achieve the healing effect.

4. It has been said above that there are five kinds of movements of the vital air. Let us see the practical aspect of this. You have been learning about *prāṇa*, that is the movement up to the plexus. Following that, you have learnt about *samāna* when you were conducting the *prāṇa* to the abdomen. Now I will explain the practice of all five at a higher level. Higher level means that after doing the initial practices described until now, you will learn to stay with the minimum requirement of the *prāṇa* energy and concentrating on that specific part out of the five said earlier. In the state of stillness, one brings oneself in perfect harmony with the *prāṇic* energy of the cosmos and one requires very little inhalation and exhalation.

   A. For *prāṇa*, concentrate on plexus and do the *prāṇāyāma* practice with both the nostrils. With a repeated practice, you will reach a state of stillness. If you are totally immersed within yourself and the chain of thoughts in the mind is hindered, your breathing process will slow down automatically.

   B. For *samāna*, you have to conduct the vital air to the navel region. All your concentration is on your navel region while you inhale and exhale and keep the *prāṇa* inside and outside. Do these four steps in a prolonged manner initially and then same thing will happen as described above. The breathing will slow down, as you are totally immersed within yourself. You are in a state of stillness and in harmony with the cosmos and your *prāṇa* is circulating in the navel region.

C. In *apāna*, you are conducting the vital air from the navel region to the feet and your concentration is on this lower region of your body. From the navel region, let the *prāṇa* energy flow to both your legs and up to your two feet. The rest of the technique is the same as described above.

D. In *udāna*, the direction of the vital air is upwards towards your head. At initial stages, when you inhale, let the *prāṇa* circulate in all parts of your head. Then bring your concentration on the totality of your head and slow down the breathing.

E. In *vyāna*, while you inhale, let the *prāṇa* energy circulate in whole of your body. Do it in a systematic manner. First take it to the plexus and then let it go towards head and arms. Then go from plexus through the navel region to the lower back and then in two directions towards both your legs and feet. It all seems so long from the description but at the subtle level with *prāṇa* energy, this journey of the whole body is done very rapidly.

You should repeatedly practice these five methods to regulate the movement of *prāṇa* in whole of your body so that you can use them for the purpose of healing the affected parts at the time of need.

Programme number twelve

Some practical aspects of prāṇāyāma

In this programme, I will describe some *prāṇāyāma* practices, which can be used for immediate benefit in specific situations. But I repeat once again that you should not practice these unless you have a mastery over the previously described techniques. With the greed of obtaining benefit from the following methods, if you force yourself to do these, you may harm yourself. On the other hand, if you are well experienced in *prāṇāyāma*, you can do the following practices with ease and can achieve successful results for your well-being.

1. To release tension or to get rid of a situation, which makes you feel sad or depressed, do the following practice. Sit

down in a comfortable position, preferably cross-legged. Inhale gradually but to your full capacity. Keep the air inside you for about seven seconds and then take it out in the form of whistling by curling your lips in about three times. That means, do not bring out all the air at once but give two stops in between. In fact, after having stopped the air for seven seconds inside you, it will gush out if you are not well versed in the *prāṇāyāma* techniques. This technique should be used only if you have enough ability to do it after a repeated practice of controlling the breath. In case you force yourself, you may get a headache.

2. To produce heat in your body in case you are feeling cold and your hands and feet get cold in winter, do the following practice. This practice is essentially the same as described in Programme seven, step 3 except that in this you forcibly hold the breath inside you. Close one of the nostrils and inhale through the other to your full capacity. Close both the nostrils as has been told earlier and keep the breath inside you as long as you get heat in all parts of your body. It means, keep the breath more than your capacity of keeping it inside. Then exhale it through the other nostril gradually. This practice is quite difficult to do, as the breath kept inside very long will gush out. A repeated practice is needed to attain mastery.
3. For getting over the feeling of hunger or thirst, make a sound with your throat while your mouth is closed. With this method, some air is produced in your mouth. Take this air inside you as if you are drinking water. That means in small quantities, you gulp it down into your throat. If you do this practice too many times, you may get a bloating feeling in your stomach. Therefore, in the beginning, do only a few times. In case you get the feeling of an over-filled stomach, do the whole body posture as shown in Figure 35.

CHAPTER 4

Prevention and Cure of Ailments

Some of you may find this chapter very attractive and may like to read it before the rest of the book. You may do so. But it is not possible to take advantage of the methods I have described here for saving you from ailments, before you put into practice what I have earlier instructed. Unfortunately, nothing is free, all has a price in one form or the other. We have to work to get all in life. If we get something free, it is because somebody else has worked for us. In the present context, with the help of a good teacher, your task may be made easier. But in any case, to use the following methods to get rid of some of the ailments, you need some training and application of the previously described wisdom. I will take here some fundamental aspects of prevention and cure and take few examples of some ailment. If you do not find your specific problem you are trying to handle, you may look into my other books. For more complex problems, you may need a private holistic physician who can guide you with what to deal first and how.

Before you begin to use these methods for prevention and cure, recall yourself the holistic concepts once again and try to forget as much as you can that your body works like a machine and can be split into different fragments for diagnostic and curative purposes. Modern way of living is fragmented and we get brainwashed by it. It needs some mental training to realise, live and feel the comic oneness at a conscious level by an individual. What I wish to remind you in the present context is that each cell of your body is a cosmos by itself. It is alive, it has its own organisation and is capable of synthesising and destroying things, communicating with other cells and performing infinite number of other functions. It has five elements, *vāta, pitta* and *kapha* perform its functions and it has the radiance of the soul and the *prāṇa* energy in it. No doubt that different organisms of our body (made of several individual cells) are designed to perform specific functions, but this performance is not a mechanical process the way we are generally taught in biology classes and medical colleges. All our parts are interconnected with blood vessels, nerves and lymphatic vessels. These not only carry the products for exchange but also have subtle communication network that we do not understand in the laboratory. I can present my views only in the form of a theory. Memory is not limited to brain but all parts of the body also store it in some subtle or elemental form. Peripheral nervous system is the extension of central nervous system, but the peripheral nervous system also sends its messages to the central nervous system and these affect our thought process and our personality. It means harmony or disturbance in any part or organ of the body is communicated to the neurons and in central nervous system, it is spread everywhere. Thus, we can take advantage of this communication in a positive manner in spreading harmony through our bodily efforts to the mind and through mental efforts to the body. I have been preparing you in the previous chapters for the formation of basic tools for this purpose. These are the mastery over body with *āsanas*, mastery over mind with self-discipline, restraint and abstinence and *prāṇāyāma*.

Tension, stress and worries

These three are ailments by themselves as well as they are the root cause of many disorders and that is why I am taking this problem at first. In the beginning, tension etc. may cause you some minor disorders which may come and go but if they continue to pest you or you let them do so, they may become causative factor for a big disease or an incurable disorder.

Tension and stress can be created in both body and mind individually or together whereas worry's domain is mind. But it is not limited to mind–it generates tension in one way or the other in the whole body and causes various *vāta*-related disorders like sleeplessness, constipation, dry throat, loss of appetite and so on. As far as tension is concerned, we may get it in mind to begin with and then we may get a stiff neck, shoulders etc. We may also create tension in one of our body parts, for example, if we sit too long in the same posture and do that very often. This happens in working situations with most people and I have discussed this theme at length in my Āyurveda book on work efficiency (*Sixteen Minutes to a Better 9-to-5*). I will give just one example here–that is of desk workers who generally get problems with stomach and digestion because there is too much physical stress on the plexus region with the result of sitting too long. Just with the physical stress, the organism may begin mal-functioning because it is squeezed in space and thus lacks one of the fundamental elements— ether. Even if you are over-worked and do not have time to stand and do bending-backward *āsana* as described in the previous Chapter, you may bend backward from time to time while sitting.

I have done research on the problem of tension and have found out that many people store tension in one of the specific body organs. If we study the proverbs in different languages, we find that they reveal ancient wisdom, which we have forgotten in modern times. My ideas is to make you aware of different case studies so that you start observing yourself in that light and than are able to handle your specific case.

Before I go into the details of this matter, I want to bring across to you that the tension we store in a body organ or a body part may or may not be related to our thought process. For example, when some people hear a bad news or there is an event that may not have good consequences in future and so on, they may have an immediate reaction to relieve themselves. It is not that body reacts because of mental tension. Actually, the event has an effect both on our body and mind simultaneously. In fact, the physiological process of excretion is in a way an outlet for this tension.

Awareness programme for detecting tension

I will give you certain possible situations, which may cause tension in diverse parts of the body. This sort of tension, if it happens too often, may become a habit. The purpose of giving you these situations is to make you aware of your own situations and your own body, which may also react in similar situations. Once you have identified that, you should try to do some concentration practices by living that situation in your thoughts. During this process of concentration, you will be able to identify the parts of the body that get tense.

Situation one: You have a meeting in one hour's time and before that you have to finish certain amount of work. You are doing well but there is a little fear in your mind. You have to find out which part of your body gets tense in this situation. There are possibilities of legs, neck, shoulders or wrists getting tense. The idea of having to go as soon as the work finishes may put the legs in some indirect position of attention because movement is their function.

Situation two: You are going to bed, you have to get up early the next day and therefore you have short night. You want to sleep immediately in order to get enough rest and this hurry gives you tension. Possible place of tension is the head region, specifically, the area around the eyebrows.

Situation three: This is a general habit with many people to make their forehead, muscle around their mouth or shoulders tense specially when they are conversing with others. Some get a frown, the others get vertical lines on the forehead and there are others who get lines above and under their lips. This tension is also transferred in the surrounding areas of those regions. Therefore, keep a constant check on yourself and massage these parts to relax them.

Situation four: If you have to solve many problems on the telephone and it gets too much for you to hear those unpleasant things which bring tension, your ears may react to it. You may get whistling, throbbing and irritation in them. It is generally the right ear that makes problems as most of us put the receiver with the right hand on the right ear. The tension of the ear is associated with the ringing of the telephone.

There are hundreds of situations like that and it is not useful to give you so much text. The message is that beware and if you have signs of pain or stiffness even in the remotest parts of your body like thumbs, toes and so on, think of this that you may be storing tension in these parts.

Tension originating from frustration

The tension of this category is even more dangerous than the above-described. The frustration in many life situations like in family life, professional life and so on slowly enters into your being; generally it attacks that part of your body which is weak by nature or it accumulates in the organ related to that action. If you do not create a timely balance, it acquires the form of a disease. For example, the accumulated tension due to frustration with a partner may give rise to diseases of uterus, breasts and prostate. Professional frustration may cause some mental ailments whereas the frustration at work place may result in severe aches or paralysis. Methods of Āyurvedic yoga are unable to help you when the serious disease is already there. That is why, it is very essential to be aware of all these possible dangers of tension and keep fighting against them constantly. Always remember that when you are at the prime of your youth, let us say between 21 and 45 years, your body can withstand the effect of negative factors but nevertheless it does not forget the harm you do to it. The older you are, the lesser your resistance becomes in every respect and you are more vulnerable to harm yourself with tension and other health-ruining activities. Therefore, one should get into the habit of settling negative accounts with the positive *sattvic* factors.

Methods to fight back the ill effects of tension

With a regular practice of *prāṇāyāma* and *yogāsanas,* you are able to develop an intuitive wisdom with which you can make the exact diagnosis of your source of tension and its ill effect on you. With constant awareness and alertness and with Āyurvedic yoga, you can succeed in uprooting the problems from the beginning. Let me explain to you all this with a concrete example. Supposing you have pain in your right shoulder. You diagnose the tension and realise that after working, you still keep your arm in 'working condition'. That means after carrying a bag with the right hand, you continue to maintain posture of tension. If you have a hectic day when you were on the move the whole day and were also carrying a bag, you realise that even at night you maintain that tense posture as if you are carrying weight. What will help is to check this situation all the time and train yourself to relax the concerned organ. The method of relaxation is to let the tense part loose and send a few times the *prāṇa* energy into this tense part as you have learnt in the previous Chapter of this Section. Yogic posture of lying down with both the arms stretched up and with a total concentration on arms and shoulders will also be very helpful in this direction. Massage is an additional cure. But remember always that these measures will not end your problem and the pain will become chronic. The only real remedy is to get rid of the persisting tension. You should be very adamant in your pursuit and several times a day you should send your *prāṇa* energy to your shoulder and arm. Do not forget to do that before sleeping and immediately after getting up. Such pains usually increase after sleeping because the tension is maintained during sleep. With the *prāṇic* exercises before going to bed, you will get rid of this tension.

If you suffer from familial or professional tension, either change your situation or protect yourself by building a protective covering or *kavaca* around you. The technique of making a *kavaca* will be described in the next Chapter. You also need considerable amount of detachment to continue to live in an unhappy situation if you wish that this unhappiness does not affect you. We have already discussed this theme of detachment earlier in the book.

What is stress?

There is a need to discuss this term as there are many different meanings attached to it. Some say it is a kind of pressure on you to finish a task or achieve something and certain degree of it is good for work efficiency. I do not agree with this opinion at all and I believe that stress is a state of helplessness when you see yourself with no escape but only with one way. If this given way does not work, you visualise either a catastrophe or a situation of extreme shamefulness or something which you do not even want to think about or imagine. There is no doubt that a stress situation may make some of you achieve your goal but the consequent results of undergoing stress frequently may affect your digestion, blood circulation, heart, arteries, brain and virtually everything in your body. Therefore, in my opinion stress should be avoided and with *sattva* one should enhance one's efficiency and get rid of stress. I have described many methods to this effect in my book, *Sixteen Minutes to a Better 9-to-5.* With tranquillity and inner stillness, one can achieve much more than with stress. Stress closes the creative faculties of the mind and the quality of work diminishes. Therefore live and work with no stress but with *Śānti* (peace and harmony).

Stress basically is linked to the limitation of time or limitation of capability. Sometimes the limitation of both is causing stress. Stress is caused constantly in some people's lives. These are the people who say that they have to work with deadlines. There are others who face stress situations from time to time either due to their own chaotic way of working or working with organisations which are not systematic and efficient or merely due to circumstances. Sometimes there are multiple factors like sickness, other unexpected difficulties of life, natural calamities and so on. Children undergo tremendous amount of stress mostly because adults impose their own ways and thinking on them whereas children behave and act in a spontaneous and natural way. This stress begins from the babies as their silent language is not heard most of the time and they are fed and taken care of as the adults have decided to do. Same is the case with their education. Anyhow, this theme is very elaborate and will be handled in my forthcoming book on children.

How to deal with stress?

Seven basic methods to deal with stress

1. Basically, stress should be dealt with **anti-stress wisdom**, as stress is fundamentally a state of mind. During stress situation the nature of the mind or *cittavṛtti,* (*Yogasūtra,* Part I, Sūtra 2) is oriented to be pressurised with fear and confusion. Yoga is all about developing the ability to change one's *cittavṛtti* and I have given several methods during the course of this book, which teach you how to stop your chain of thoughts. As soon as we stop the chain of thoughts, the confusion and fear vanish and clarity comes. The quick method to attain inner calm in stress situation is to direct *prāṇa* energy to your head region; hold it there and let it out gradually by releasing all your stress. Whenever fear, anguish or confusion prevails, take recourse to *prāṇāyāma* immediately.
2. Try to apply the wisdom we have been discussing in the last chapter on **detachment**, greed etc. in your specific case. Remember always you are not the creator of other people's destiny and for your own, you will do the best by staying calm.
3. Sometimes one has suddenly too many things going wrong in one's life. This gives the feeling of helplessness, oppression and stress. Remember always that such happenings are a part of one's life. It is not only you who are undergoing bad times. All of us have to go through various good or bad situations in our life. We tend to take good and happy events of life for granted and we usually do not express our gratefulness. We take painful happenings as if a special torture is being inflicted on us. We are harvesting the fruits of our *karma.* Keep doing things for the well-being of others even when you have distressed times. Remember Patañjali's Sūtra 15 of Part II where he states that **even happiness is pain for the wise** as it never lasts forever and its departure

is painful. Thus the real method to fight out stress lies in doing a constant training of one's mind to stay stable both in good and bad times. Different offshoots of yoga, the *Bhagavadgītā* and the Vedas including Āyurveda convey this basic message of keeping one's balance in both happy and unhappy states.

4. There is the **stress of big cities,** which all of us have to face. With so many vehicles, traffic jams, pollutants and crowds, this stress takes a toll on us with time. Our power of discerning and intellect diminish with a constant stress like that. We as individuals cannot save ourselves totally from it if we happen to have our home or work in one of these big metropolises, but there is some part of stress that we can still manage. That is done by **learning to withdraw** oneself from the crowds. Bring all your thoughts to your own self and concentrate on the energy that is the cause of your being, the soul.
5. You should cultivate the habit of **living in the present moment** of time. It is the time we are living in that is the most important. In fact, stress is a state of mind that is generally engulfed in the fear of the future. If you save your energy from this fear, you can utilise it in a positive manner and be more efficient and successful in whatever you are doing. Do not take things so terribly seriously. Save your life and health from this poison called stress. Imagine that you are a pilot and you have to fly a plane with 300 persons aboard to some far off destination. You are stuck in worst ever traffic jam and are getting late for your flight. This is quite a serious situation that can cause a considerable amount of stress. But you are really helpless and there is nothing you can do to make the situation better. Try to console yourself by saying that this trouble I am undergoing is better than any bigger trouble like having an accident. This method you should always try to apply in diverse situations. If one imagines that things could have been even worse, the present situation becomes more tolerable.
6. This method is **ritualistic.** If you feel suddenly oppressed by a situation and feel completely helpless, then perform this little ritual. Stand straight, close your eyes and visualise your whole body. Raise both your hands and keep them at

a little distance from your face and go around with them from front to top to back of your head. Repeat that three times. Do also three times on the front part of your body and then at the neck and back as far as your hands can reach. Now use left hand to go around the right arm and shoulder and vice versa. Bend down a little and move both your hands first around the right leg and feet and then around the left leg and feet (Figures 43-46). Come back to the straight position and think of the solar energy. Imagine the form of the Sun between your two eyebrows,

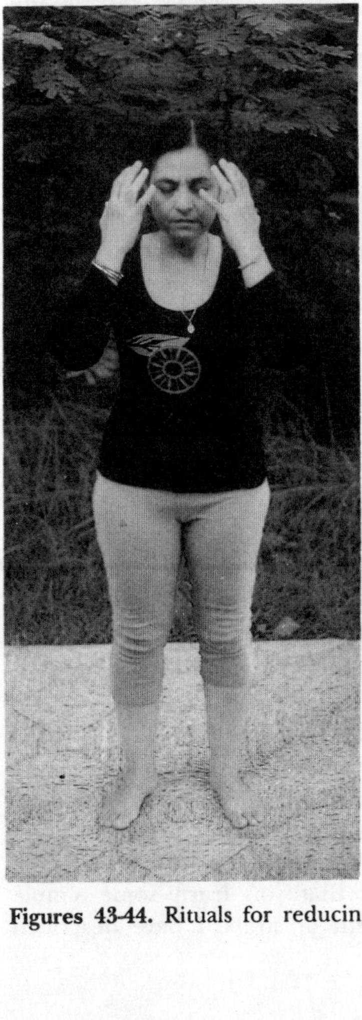

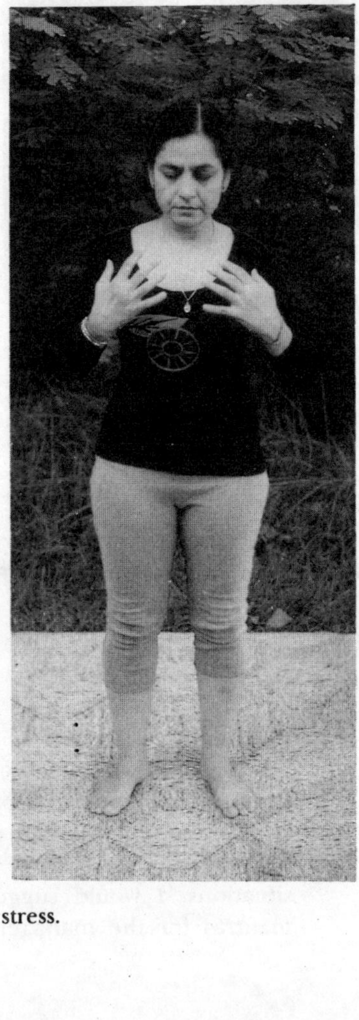

Figures 43-44. Rituals for reducing stress.

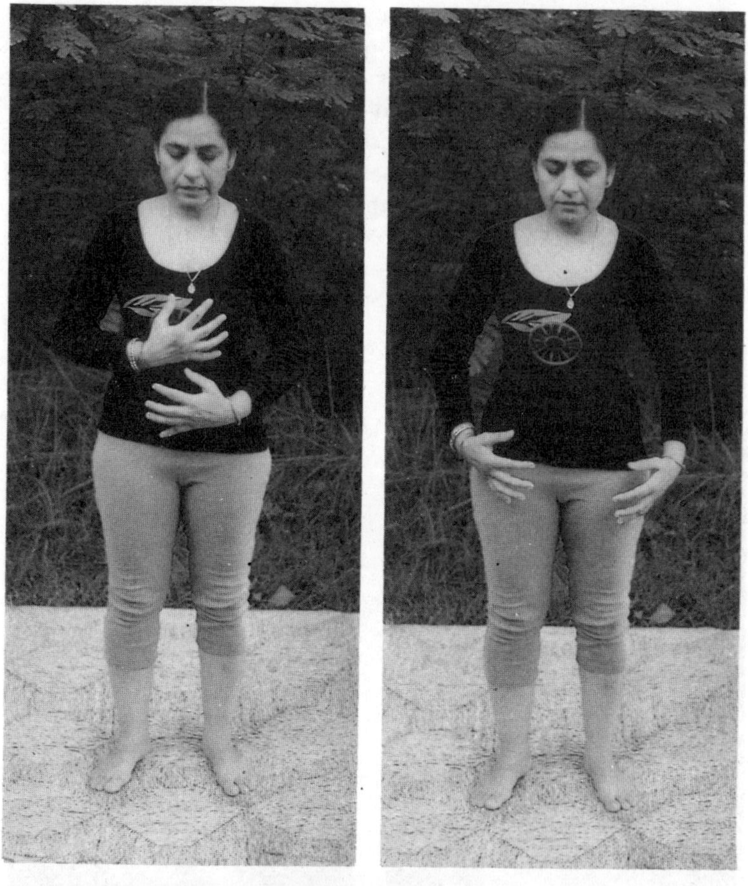

Figures 45-46. Rituals for reducing stress.

practice *prāṇāyāma* with subdued breathing and feel the energy of the Sun within you. His light will show you the right path and help you solve your problems, which are causing stress.

7. In traditional Hindu families, we are taught the yogic practices of concentration and *japa* etc. from the very beginning. These are a part of religious and ceremonious Hindu tradition. Mantras play a special role in our lives and provide us strength. We learn mantras for various life situations. I would suggest that you learn some simple mantras for the management of stress. I have described

some simplified mantras in my previous books. You may choose according to your situation. Otherwise, you may also invent your own themes for mantras. For example, you may repeat the name of a strong tree or a mountain to get strength and face the difficult period when you feel oppressed with life situations. Developing a link with some natural power which is close to your surroundings like a lake, river or an old tree etc. is another way of getting strength. You may visualise one of these at the time of need.

Stress and modern technology

It is interesting that every body talks of stress related to modern technology, enhanced pace of life, too much traffic and so on. But we also must remember that technology has also helped us to lessen our stress. With enhanced pace of communication, cellular phones, fax, Internet etc. life has become easier. In ancient times also, people used to travel between Europe and India and they were travelling for months to reach their destinations. Their families had no way of communicating with them. In our times, we have the privilege of travelling from Delhi to Frankfurt in less than eight hours.

Worries

Many people create lot of health problems for themselves because they worry too much. Worry never brings anything positive, neither for the problem you are worrying about nor for the people about whom you worry. By worrying, one has a negative chain of thoughts. With strength of yogic methods, you must learn to break this chain of thoughts and bring stillness to your mind. Worry can give you many mental ailments as well as heart, liver or other related disorders. It can throw your metabolism out of gear and your humours out of balance. You may get diabetes, colitis, stomach ulcers and number of other terrible health disorders. In Hindi, a proverb puts it very strongly—*cintā citā samāna* (Worry is like a funeral pyre).

If you have learnt the basic yogic capability of stopping the chain of thoughts, you can free yourself from this evil of worrying. But the problem is that some people do not realise that to worry is destructive and prepares ground for ailments. They, in a way, feel important that they have so many worries. I feel that when people are older and their children are grown up, worry is sometimes a means to get rid of loneliness. By worrying about their adult children, the parents indirectly feel as if they in a way still live with them. I suggest that you should find better vocation for yourself than worry.

People generally worry because they are afraid that future may not be according to what they expect. If they continue to worry, the future will certainly not be as they expect because they will be sick. Instead of worrying about yourself, about your dear ones and about the fears of future related to sickness, accident, natural calamities etc. put your *sattvic* thoughts in warding off bad events.

Some suggestions for warding off worries

If you are convinced that worrying does not mend matters, I am sure you can stop worrying. Following are some constructive suggestions to bring *sattvic* thoughts into your mind to replace worry and to be constructive rather than destructive.

1. Many people worry about **getting sick with a serious incurable disease like cancer, AIDS** etc. I suggest that instead make a **prayer** on getting up in the morning to the Sun to protect you from disease and give you long life. Do also your concentration exercises before going to bed so that you have *yoganidrā* or *sattvic* sleep rather than *rajasic* and *tamasic* sleep full of action and worries. These prayers are in addition to living in a holistic way for good health and harmony.
2. If you are worried about **accidents** while travelling or when your dear ones are travelling, start saying **special prayers to ether, air and sun** for an obstruction—free travel at least 15 days before the proposed travelling and during the travelling. When you return home safely, say the prayers of gratefulness to these three elements. Ether and air are the elements for movements and sun is for showing you the way.
3. If you are worried about **not being able to finish a project** within a given time limit, or something alike, your special demands of success should be addressed to ***Kāla*—Time**. In such situations, the Hindus address their prayers to goddess *Kāli*—the goddess that personifies time.
4. If you are worried about your dear ones who have **trouble**

in one way or the other, **do mantras and concentration exercises** for their well being. Make a **protective armour (*kavaca*)** around them every now and then and keep sending mentally your good wishes to them. It is made by inhaling and sending the *prāṇa* energy to the plexus and covering your entire body in it while you exhale this energy out from the plexus region. This is the region where the soul resides and it is the most vital area of our body.

5. After having studied Patañjali, you know that when we break the chain of thoughts and stop the thinking process, the mind identifies itself with the soul—the immense source of energy that is beyond space and time. At that state, there is no worry but only **inner joy or *ānanda*.** Therefore, try the concentration exercises described in this book and take the worrying mind to the realms of beatitude.

If you make an effort to replace your worrying habits with *sattvic* thoughts, you will find yourself a changed person and at peace with yourself.

Methods to enhance memory

In Sūtra 11 of Part I, Patañjali defines memory as, 'Memory is the retention of notion one has had'. Memory can be both afflictive and non-afflictive. Some people keep thinking about the past either to appreciate it and feel unhappy that the good times are gone or to pity themselves that they have gone through terrible suffering in their lives. There are others who can never get over their bad childhood and keep blaming their parents for all the ills in their lives. In all these cases, it is afflictive use of memory. I wish to teach you some methods of enhancing memory for constructive use. My purpose is that you should promote your memory not only for attaining success in your profession but also to remember always to do your yogic practices, to begin your day and night with *sattvic* thoughts, to remember not to worry and to remember to get rid of the stress.

I come in contact with many people who complain that they have problems with their memory and they suffer from forgetfulness. But on examination, mostly it turns out to be that it is not their memory which has problem but they are not paying attention. This can be easily found out as such persons are capable of narrating certain incidents of their liking or some sensational events in amazing details and they are far from any memory loss in biological or medical terms.

In our times, when many people consume very anti-peace nonsense from the media with images which last only a fraction of a second and so on, the attention span becomes very little. They become incapable of listening to you carefully and retaining what you have said. Hence, many times, there is distortion of reality. The methods of yoga can be used to enhance attentiveness, concentration and memory. I am giving below some simple suggestions and exercises that will help you to enhance your retention capabilities. For those of you, who do creative work, it will be very beneficial to use the yogic method of *dhyāna*.

1. Remember always that *rajas*ic and *tamasic* thoughts enhance forgetfulness and loss of memory. In fact, these qualities make a cover of darkness to reproduce the information already retained in mind. Do your morning and evening exercises regularly and practice *prāṇāyāma* as a way of life as has been told earlier. This will bring stillness of mind that enhances attention span and retention power.
2. Talking too much and being in noisy environment diminish memory. Make an effort to talk less, find some quiet moments each day when you can be on your own. Do not talk before going to bed and immediately after getting up. One should slowly glide into the quietness of night and should gradually come to the wakeful state with the light of the day.
3. When you forget something, which you urgently need to recall, do not panic. The moment you panic, your recalling capacity is even more depressed. Be quiet and keep confidence in your mental faculty. Send *prāṇa* energy to your head a few times but not with the idea that you are trying to recall something. After that, try to concentrate on the form of the thing you are looking for or something related to the incident you are trying to recall. If you are able to break the chain of thoughts and concentrate fully on the theme or the subject, you will certainly have success.
4. If you do not get enough and appropriate sleep, you may develop the problems of forgetfulness. Make every effort to get *sattvic* sleep or *yoganidrā* as has been described in the

previous Chapter.

5. If you have *vāta* imbalance, which persists too long, it affects your nerves and memory. You become nervous, hectic in your mannerisms and forgetful. If this is the situation, take appropriate measures with inner cleaning practices and medication to get rid of *vāta* imbalance.
6. All yogic *āsanas* where feet are lifted upwards and blood flow is directed towards the head are memory promoting. Needless to say that all the concentration practices—*japa, dhyāna* etc. are memory promoting. They not only help us recall the events of the past of this life but also of our past lives which we have within us in the form of *saṃskāra*. As has been mentioned earlier, *saṃskāra* are a kind of memory over a broader dimension of time.
7. I will describe here what I call the **RECALLING EXERCISES**, which are very beneficial to enhance memory. These exercises are very simple. Before going to bed, try to recall in a sequence a part of your day. You may choose any part of your day. Next day, upon getting up in the morning, try to recall another part of the day. The recalling should be in sequence and in details of what all you did during those 2-3 hours you are trying to recall. This exercise is also done on a larger time scale. Try to recall an event or a specific day that you had lived ten years ago. This exercise should be repeated for ten to fifteen days trying to recall the same incident and the happenings around it. You will see that this exercise may make you recall or dream of other events of this period too. These are generally very subtle things that you think you have already forgotten. This exercise has a cleansing effect on the brain and enhances memory.

Needless to say that with all these seven suggestions, you should also take some memory promoting products, which I have described in my Āyurveda books.

Increasing the power to concentrate

The moment we concentrate on something, the chain of thoughts in our mind is stopped and all our mental energy is focussed at one single point. We all are aware that the capacity and ease to concentrate varies from one time to another. There are times when we are able to concentrate with ease whereas there are other times when our mind wanders a lot. In fact, during the process of trying to concentrate our thoughts on a single point, whether this is a piece of our own work or it is for the purpose of yoga, our state of mind at that particular moment is reflected. In this respect, the mind is a mirror for itself. Thus, the more we keep our mind balanced with *sattvic* thoughts, the easier it becomes to concentrate on a subject. The more our mind is cluttered with thoughts from too many people, from speaking loud, from watching different things on television and so on, the more we have to struggle to concentrate. For learning new things, we have to concentrate. The more we keep learning, the more our mind is purified and the more we develop the ability to concentrate. In fact, one of the purposes of education is to teach us to develop our faculty to concentrate. That is the why, the more we learn, the more we develop the capability of learning. Thus, one way of learning to concentrate is- NEVER STOP LEARNING.

Sometimes, the problem of lack of concentration is temporary and it may be due to imbalance of *vāta*. If your basic nature or *prakṛti* is *vāta* and you are suffering from constipation that causes vitiation of this humour; the lack of concentration is the obvious result of that. In that case, take a *vāta* appeasing tea like a mixture of cardamom, ginger, basil, take a warm enema with camomile decoction, oil your body and take some rest. You will see that the problem of lack of concentration will not be there after taking these measures. Similarly, fast moving wind, low atmospheric pressure or sudden change in weather may give rise to this problem. Massage, warm bath, some yogic postures and *prāṇāyāma* are enough to develop the ability to concentrate.

In this case also, like in of getting rid of stress, yogic practice called *japa* of a mantra as has been described earlier is helpful. You should understand that basically in both the cases, problem is the same, you have to control your mind, stop it from wandering elsewhere and bring it where you want it to be.

Concentration is basically to train the mind to behave as directed. This can be developed with some pleasant methods like singing, playing musical instruments, taking up other performing arts and handicrafts. What exactly you take up to enhance concentration depends on the nature of your problem and factors causing it. If your lack of concentration is caused by sadness, depression or similar sentiments, it is better you take up activities which are performed in a group like singing in chorus or playing theatre. If your thoughts wander too much here and there and you are nervous and hectic, you get very quickly excited about things, then you should take up something like carving, painting, pottery etc.

As described above, a mental training of 'living in the given moment of time' also enhances the power to concentrate. If you systematically work on yourself with the earlier described exercises of keeping a check on yourself etc., then you can easily train yourself in 'living in the given moment of time'. The ability to concentrate is the key to success in all domains of life, whether your aim is material or spiritual or somewhere in the middle, which I suggest in this book.

Curing various aches and pains

The difference between physiotherapy (which is also partly inspired from yogic exercises) and curing yourself with Āyurvedic yoga is that the latter is not dealing with merely at the physical level. In Āyurvedic yoga, all treatments are done at rational, mental and spiritual levels. For curing the aches from posture defects, body imbalance, excessive use of a particular organ and so on, *āsanas, prāṇāyāma* and healing practices are done simultaneously along with the herbal and massage treatments.

While curing with Āyurvedic yoga, you should keep one thing in mind that the fundamental philosophy of yoga is to attain the aim with repeated practice and persistence (*Yogasutra,* Part I, Sūtra 12-14). In healing and curing ailments, you have to apply this basic idea. With all your might, you have to get after your trouble or imbalance. When your mental force, your physical effort, and your spiritual energy come together, it can do wonders. The healing is not be done like an instant wonder. The extent of the effort will be directly proportional to how deep the roots of the ailment are. But keep in mind that you have to have courage and get after the ailment with all your mental strength and with a repeated effort. Think of a little child who wants something (a chocolate for example) from his mother and the mother says a very stern 'NO'. The child persists, says the same in different emotions and tones and then adds superlatives to it. He/she compliments the mother for being always so good and caring and so on. In this process, the children may say something very funny that makes the mother laugh and relax. Her heart melts with the repeated persistence of her child and she ends up giving the desired thing. You should have this child-like attitude to achieve your goal in curing aches or healing other ailments.

In almost all my books on yoga and Āyurveda, I have described different methods to cure various ailments. Here I will give you some model examples so that you get a comprehensive idea and can select *āsanas* and other methods for your specific case. Please look for the details of the *āsanas* in my other books. Here, I will only refer to the name of the *āsanas.*

Menstrual pains

Many women in the world suffer every month from menstrual cramps and discomforts. I have discussed this problem in details in my book—*The Kāmasūtra for Women.* I once again want to emphasise here that you should make an effort to get rid of this perpetual problem by appropriate diet, precautions and *āsanas.* Do the salutation to the sun twelve times everyday throughout the month except at the time of menstruation. You should learn it properly with a good teacher and do these as regularly as you brush your teeth or eat your meals. When doing *āsanas* for curative purpose, the therapy should not be subjected to your having time and doing them every now and then. Their therapeutic value will be lost. Besides, for curative purpose, the *āsanas* should be done in an appropriate manner with full intentness of mind.

All those *āsanas,* which exercise your abdominal part will also be helpful in revitalising the reproductive organs and thus help to cure the cramps during menstruation.

Backaches and shoulder pains

If you do not distribute your body weight properly and you put more of your weight on left or right side of the body, you can disturb the delicate balance of the vertebrae that your back maintains and can get diverse kinds of backaches. Since this is the part where your spinal chord as well as the major blood vessels pass through and supply branches, any imbalance can cause severe pain in different parts of the back, shoulders and arms, in pelvic region and legs. I am telling you all these details just to suggest to you that even if you do not have backache or allied pains, you should do *yogāsanas* to make your back strong. In the previous Chapter, I have described some *āsanas* to make the back strong. They are very advanced *āsanas* and are not meant to be done when you already have pain. For that situation, you should do the six backbone *āsanas* I have mentioned earlier. I suggest that these backbone *āsanas* should be done by everybody (especially people who sit a lot and work) as preventive measure. There are many people whose backbone is not straight and because of that they start getting troubles in their forties. These exercises will help to keep the backbone straight and reduce the possibility of pain with aging.

Those of you who have forward bent shoulders are bound to get trouble with the upper part of the back, shoulders and even arms. Correct always your posture and in addition do the following āsana and the movements.

Lie down with your arms stretched upwards, straight and parallel to each other (Figure 47). Let your self loose and completely immerse yourself in this form of your body. Imagine an axis in the middle part of your head and a straight line going through your spine and then between your two legs and feet. Those of you who have bent shoulders will not be able to keep the arms straight—they will be lifted up from the ground. Make an effort each time to straighten them slightly more and if you

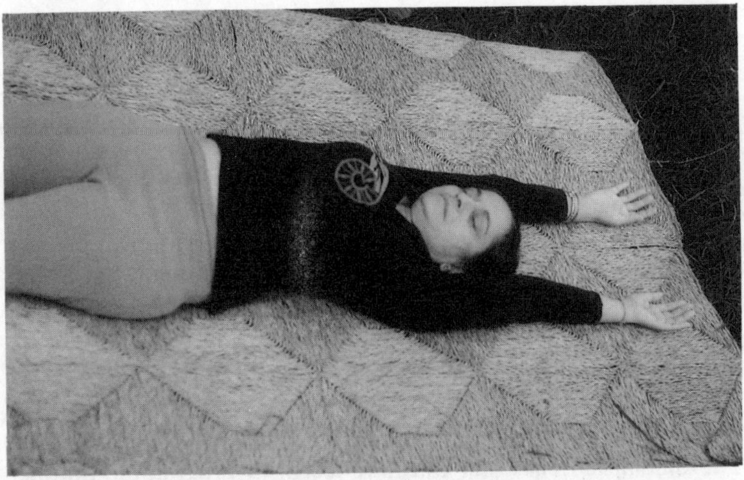

Figure 47. A supine *āsana* with arms stretched upwards.

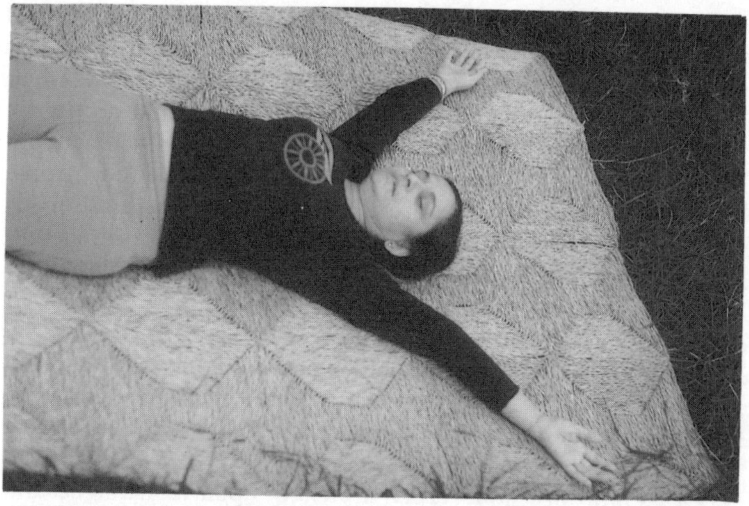

Figure 48. Making semicircles with the arms after having made the *āsana* in Figure 47.

are persistent, you will be able to cure your posture defect in six months to one year.

The next step is to make a half circle with both your arms and bring them parallel to your body (Fig. 48). Some of you may find this painful as due to bad posture, the whole area will be stiff. If this is the case, do it gradually and slowly and the stiffened muscles will relax.

Because of your bent shoulders, the upper part of your back also acquires a bent form. The vertebral column acquires an outward bent arch. Thus, the above shoulder exercises have to be combined with the six backbone exercises so that the back goes on acquiring the straight form simultaneously. If you work hard and persistently, it may take you nearly a year to cure this posture defect completely but think of all those years that you have been making this defective posture. The older you are, the longer it will take to cure but always remember it is never too late to begin good things in life.

Weakness and pain in legs and sciatica

The *uttānapādāsanas* that you have learnt in Programme number two involving lifting the leg/legs upwards are extremely beneficial to cure weakness in this part of the body as well as sciatica. In case of sciatica, you will have to take other precautions also as I have described in my book, *Āyurveda a Way of Life.* In case your legs are too weak and you are unable to do these *āsanas*, do not go too far up with lifting the leg. Make only slight up and down movements and get massages with pain relieving oils, hot baths and fomentation. All these treatments will strengthen your legs and gradually you will be able to have success in making these *āsanas.*

In addition to the four earlier described *āsanas*, I will describe one more here which you should do only when you have attained mastery over the earlier ones. Since this one requires strength from your pelvic and abdominal muscles, if you force yourself, you might get muscle cramps.

Lie down on your back with both hands slightly apart from each other. Keep both your feet also at a distance of about 20 centimetre apart from each other. Relax completely and start lifting one of your legs upwards. When this leg is at about 45°, begin lifting the other leg also. Lift them both simultaneously but they should remain at a distance from each other. When the first leg will reach at 90° angle, the second will be at 45° (Figure 49). Remain in this posture a little while and then alter the position of the legs

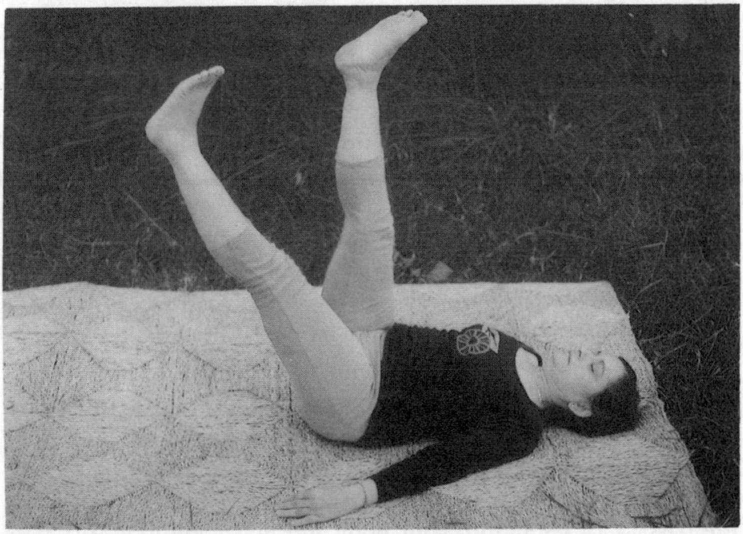

Figure 49. *Uttānapādāsana* with movements of legs.

with each other. Do this a few times. This *āsana* is not only good for legs or pelvic region but also for all the internal organs in the lower abdominal region. It is excellent to shed weight from the abdominal area.

Headaches

It is rarely that the origin of headache is head itself except in case of some head injuries or neurological disorders. Mostly headaches in otherwise healthy people originate from digestive disorders like constipation, acidity, obstructed breathing due to blocked nose, vitiation of one of the humours or due to noisy and polluted environment. Therefore, when you have a headache, try to search and remove the root cause.

Women may get headaches due to menstrual problems and they should take care to maintain the equilibrium on that front as I have described in my book, *The Kāmasūtra for Women.*

The nasal passage should be always clear and do *jalaneti* at least once a week. If you tend to get a nose block, always do inhalation from etheric oils before going to bed. You should also practice purification of the head region as I have described in my book, *Sixteen Minutes to a Better 9-to-5.*

Strengthen the head region with *prāṇa* energy and when you have an inclination of getting an attack of headache apply a mixture of etheric oils or a balm made of such oils and take some rest. Sometimes the headache is caused by intake of some foodstuff, which is antagonist to the nature of our body or is spoilt. In such cases, do not hesitate to do *jaladhauti.* Drink three glasses (500-600 ml) of salted hot water and vomit it out.

Almond or sesame oil head massage or a massage with an Āyurvedic memory promoting and nerve strengthening oil is recommended once a week.

Asthma and chronic cough

For curing asthma and chronic cough, along with other precautions, the cobra *āsana* described earlier (Figure 30) is indispensable. You should make this *āsana* in the morning as well as before going to bed as these ailments enhance during night-time.

These two ailments are directly related to *prāṇa.* They obstruct the passage of *prāṇa* into your body and make you look very pale and lifeless. Because of the obstruction of phlegm or irritation in the nasal and bronchial passages, it is not possible to do *prāṇāyāma* practices during these ailments. Therefore, you should do head cleaning practice with inhalation so that these passages are cleared and you are able to take in the *prāṇa* energy. Do inhalations with etheric oils before going to bed so that you can breathe properly during the night. You have to be very active to fight back these ailments, otherwise they become chronic and it becomes all the more difficult to get rid of them. Since they are directly related to the intake of the *prāṇa* within us, they weaken all the other functions of the body also. Therefore, you are advised to be very alert not to let these ailments enhance and threaten your life functions.

A general discussion about ailments

The theme of curing ailments is very vast and I have always dealt with it extensively in all my books. Spiritual aspect of healing will be discussed in the next Chapter. However, before closing this Chapter, I want to express some general ideas about how the ailments are born. The principal idea to discuss this is to make you aware once more about the fact that there are numerous ailments which we cause for ourselves by living in a non-holistic manner. When we do acts, which are against the nature of our body or, we may say, against the life itself, we are bound to be unwell. The living energy within us protests in one way or the other in the form of ailment or trouble. These are called the innate disorders as has been said previously. Ailments like sleep disorders, abnormal blood pressure (high or low; high blood pressure is generally termed as hypertension), various heart troubles, different kinds of headaches including migraines, different liver ailments and other digestive disorders, diabetes, haemorrhoids (piles), colitis, numerous kinds of aches and pains etc. However, when we are troubled by one or several of these innate disorders, our vitality and our immune system, called *ojas* in Āyurveda, diminishes and that makes us liable to catch the external infections, less resistant to external poisons, accidents etc. Besides that, our mental strength and capacity diminishes to face various social situations and problems and we lose our toughness and courage. It is obvious that a troubled person cannot also be a fighter in life situations. This way, we become vulnerable to external attacks and mental ailments. Thus, we fall prey to the second and third kind of disorders described in Āyurveda (see Section III).

It is observed from my study in India that the poor people generally do not suffer from the innate and mental disorders. Their principal troubles are due to the unhygienic conditions they live in and due to that they constantly suffer from water-borne disorders and other parasite infections. The patients with the above-described innate disorders generally come from the affluent sections of the society and their ailments spring principally from the following factors: *asantoṣa* (lack of contentment), malnutrition related to excessive and wrong food and lack of movements and physical labour. This is the state of affairs also in other affluent societies all over the world. Āyurvedic yoga can provide a solution to these problems and can help prevent numerous innate disorders and lessen other disorders too.

CHAPTER 5

The 'Living' in the Body

In this last Chapter of the book, I am going to take up that aspect of Āyurvedic yoga, which deals with the subtle energy of the body and teaches us methods to channelise this energy for the beneficial purpose. It has been already discussed in details that the cause of consciousness is the soul and that is what brings life in the body made of five elements. When the soul enters the body and the body becomes living, then it is conscious and active and requires vital force to perform different functions. The five elements of the body make three major vital forces—*vāta, pitta* and *kapha* to perform all its functions. The energy, which keeps the body and the soul together and is our constant link with the cosmos, is *prāṇa,* which we constantly take from the atmosphere in the form of our breathing. We have talked about *prāṇa* at length in the earlier part of the book. Each part of our body is living and each cell is very actively performing its functions. In some cases, the old cells die and new cells replace them. Degeneration and regeneration are a part of the activities of the living body to maintain its equilibrium with optimum functional activity.

The living body is a complete natural system by itself, which is connected to other natural systems of the cosmos and is dependent upon them in functional, subtle and philosophical aspects. If we interfere too much with this connection and interdependence, we cause vitiation of its functions and this is what one aspect of our ailments is. Let me make my statement more explicit by giving a very simple example. During summer and monsoons in India, it is very hot—first the dry heat and then the wet heat. Nature provides us with some bitter vegetables and fruits during these seasons. They are very good to fight the heat and they also purify the blood and act as disinfectant against the waterborne ailments during the monsoons. Fruits of neem and bitter gourd are good examples in this context. If we do not eat them according to the requirements of the weather and climatic conditions, we may fall prey to one of the monsoons' ailments. On the other hand, if we try to grow these fruits and vegetables in winter with artificial climatic conditions and also consume them in winter, we may do harm to ourselves. We may end up feeling colder and may get low blood pressure due to the lack of heat and energy in our body.

As has been said in the earlier part of the book, the entire cosmos is a dynamic whole where everything is in constant movement and interaction. After having read Patañjali and introduction to *Sāṃkhya,* you may have gathered that at the time of death, the five elements of the body go back to their main pool as the body in the present state is a temporary entity and the soul is eternal. The soul is reborn later and acquires another body. As the soul enters again in the combination of ovum and sperm, the *prāṇa* and the vitality comes and the complete body is formed from the embryo.

My idea to give you a brief summary of all that what we have already dealt with in one way or the other during the course of this book is to prepare you for an understanding of the subtle energy in our body. I have already talked about it briefly in the introductory chapter but now we will go more in finer details. The aim is to understand first and then learn the techniques and ability to channelise this energy. I will gradually make you understand the concept of the subtle energy through your own experiences. The major problem is that with the materialistic and reductionist approach of the modern science and medicine, people are used to seeing everything in concrete material values. They are very much impressed by laboratory analysis, X-rays' reproductions and ultra sound etc. Indeed, these analyses are wonderful and allow us to peep in our bodies. But they are not cure or treatment. They should lead to these but it is not always possible. For using the therapeutic methods described in this book, you need to get away a little from the analysis of your body at the material level and learn to feel your inner rhythm. The methods of purification as well as *yogāsanas* and *prāṇāyāma* practices are preparatory for the purpose of a journey within one's body.

Cosmos in the smallest unit

As already said above, each cell is capable of performing numerous functions. The more we know about the cells, the more we realise that we are ignorant about them. There are a large variety of the specialised cells in our body for performing specific functions. Then we come to the interaction and the inter-communications between these cells. All this makes the task about cell knowledge exceedingly difficult. I can go on with this theme because of being a research scientist for twenty years and studying various aspects of cell structures and functions with highly developed technology. But my idea of telling you this is to make you understand that even in our times, we are only reaffirming the conclusions the sages reached in India thousands of years ago. Each cell of our body is a cosmos by itself. The sages reached this conclusion perhaps by observing nature and through meditation but it is wonderful that in our times, we can say the same thing after having experienced this phenomenon at the sensuous level with the help of high technology.

Coming to our present context of Āyurvedic yoga, each cell has five elements, the soul and the *prāṇa* energy which keeps them together. We as individuals are the bigger extension of millions of these small units. The smallest unit has also the five subtle elements, the five senses in some form or the other and of course all the five kinds of activities (see Table 2 for details of the analysis of the cosmos in *Sāṃkhya* thought).

Journey inside the body

In the totality of the bodily system, all these cells are interconnected and interdependent. There is a link in all which makes the pieces into an entirety. At this point, we are not talking of the physiological link at a material level but of energy link which binds them together. This is what makes the subtle body within the material body of arteries, veins, lymph and nerves. These energy links are made of the energy radiating from the soul and the *prāṇa*. Thus, each cell of our body has a part of that eternal energy soul and is linked with the cosmos with *prāṇa* energy. Soul is the cause of being and *prāṇa* makes the link between soul and the material reality and thus makes the performance of all the functions possible.

In the present context, the aim is to develop the ability to reach each and every part of the body through its fine energy system. This aim is achieved by establishing a connection with the energy of the soul and with *prāṇa*. *Prāṇa* is what makes the energy of the soul travel in each and every molecule of our body. As said already, *prāṇa* is the link between the body and the soul and it keeps them together. When *prāṇa* leaves the body, the soul departs and there is death. Death is not only at an individual level and for the totality of the being but also at a minute and partial scale. That means when the *prāṇa* energy is not supplied in an appropriate manner, the vital functions are subdued because the energy of the soul is covered by *tamas.* This can be true of a part of the body or an individual. Thus, the journey into the body will be basically through *prāṇa,* which will be used to illuminate oneself with the energy of the soul and enhance one's vitality. For this purpose, knowledge of *prāṇāyāma* is very essential. That is what forms the basis to reach the energy points of the body as well as channelising this energy to the other parts of the body.

From Patañjali's *Yogasūtra,* it is already clear that certain distinct points in the body have specific energy and can be used for achieving a specific goal. In Part III, Sūtra 29, it is said that by performing *saṃyama* on the circle of the navel, one can acquire the knowledge of the bodily systems. To get rid of hunger and thirst, the *saṃyama* is performed on the pit of the throat (Sūtra 30). The stability is acquired by performing *saṃyama* on the tube below the pit of the throat (Sūtra 31). The knowledge about the activities of the mind is acquired by performing *saṃyama* on *hṛdaya* or plexus (Sūtra 34).

Later in the Tantric tradition, the energy points were systematised and the anatomy of the subtle body was developed. As you see in Table 5, in the first Chapter of this book, all the energy points are thoroughly studied and their relationship with the cosmic energy is well established. From these energy points or cakras, there emerge the other finer *nāḍis* or channels which reach each and every part of the body. In the present context of the Āyurvedic yoga, we will not go in the details of the anatomy of the subtle body as has been described in Tantric tradition. For our purpose of health and healing, we will stick to two major points given by Patañjali—the navel circle and the plexus. These two will help us to diagnose the state of the body and the mind and help us to know our being in six dimensions (*vāta-pitta-kapha* and *sattva-rajas-tamas*). From these two points, with the help of *prāṇic* energy, we can reach each and every part of the body. As I have mentioned above, *prāṇa* makes the connection between the subtle and the material and thus, the subtle is not too far away from the material and the way to reach the both should be easy. My statement will be clearer when I describe later in this Chapter, Suśruta's concept of *marma.*

The purpose of the journey

This Chapter is called 'The "living" in the body' and above I have dealt with the theme of 'Journey inside the body'. Now, let us see what is the purpose of this journey. The aim of this journey is to discover this living aspect and rejuvenate it.

1. *Avoid partial death*

If we treat our body like a mechanical system and live with the thought that when something is wrong with it, it is the physician who is supposed to care for it, gradually we attain, what I call 'partial death'. That means that we are living and performing all our duties and functions but not to the optimum level. We live with a kind of feeling like 'things could be better' both physically and mentally. The lack of living each moment of life with the consciousness of living and just go on surviving may give rise to various pains and aches and other troubles which may not be life-threatening but nagging. Because of being indifferent and insensitive to the vital functions of the body, we may create imbalance and thus suffer from being constantly unwell. Thus, one of the purposes of the journey inside the body is to be able to live completely to our optimum capacity in every respect of our being and avoid 'partial death'. The purpose of the techniques given in the following programmes is to make it possible for you to detect any problem in this direction and teach you to develop the ability to 'irrigate' your body or some particular organs with energy.

2. *Enhance the 'living' element in you*

We possess infinite internal energy, which lies within us untapped. You have studied in the *Yogasūtra* how a yogī can enhance his/her capabilities and attain *siddhis.* An ordinary human being probably does not want to go as far to attain *siddhis.* But what is extremely beneficial for our everyday life is to enhance our vitality and through concentration practices and *prāṇāyāma* increase our energy and capability. It is up to us how we use this energy—for attaining sensuous pleasures or for the fulfilment of other goals. The principal point to understand is that despite our limitations as human beings due to our previous karmic conditions, all of us have equality in one respect i.e. that we have the similar capabilities of exploring the abundant energy within us with our personal efforts.

3. *Rejuvenate yourself*

One of the purposes of the journey within your body through *prāṇa* is to rejuvenate yourself. One needs rejuvenation when one has excessive physical or mental strain or due to the process of aging, one feels that the energy is diminishing. In Āyurveda, one out of the eight parts is devoted to the subject of rejuvenation. Rejuvenation with the *prāṇic* energy should be accompanied by the other methods described in Āyurveda, particularly the intake of the rejuvenating products.

4. *For healing yourself*

As said already, the journey within ourselves helps us to diagnose ourselves and through that we can know if a particular part of our body is weak. We can send the *prāṇic* energy to that part and enhance the healing process.

5. *For enhancing mental capabilities, creativity and intuitive wisdom*

All of us have much larger potentials within us than we are aware of. They lie subdued within us. With the methods of exploring ourselves, we can trap these resources within us. All the three things mentioned here are in fact in one category and they are achieved simultaneously when we silence our mind and explore it with the medium of *prāṇic* energy.

Oneness with the dynamic cosmos

I have already stated in details about the interrelationship and interdependence in all that exists in the cosmos. We all know that we are related, connected and dependent on the five elements of nature as we are a part of them in the composite form along with the soul and the *prāṇa* within us. We can use these latter two for taking direct energy from the five elements. In the following programme, there are some very simple exercises and you may make them as part of your everyday life. These methods will provide you with instant and constant vitality and your mind will get a regular practice of silencing itself.

Programme number thirteen

Receiving the cosmic energy

The methods of receiving the energy from the five elements and the other cosmic bodies is based on concentrating upon them by looking at them or by bringing their image in your mind. These methods will also help you build a relationship with your surroundings. A relationship is built with exchange and communication. Our surroundings do have a relationship with us but until we develop also the similar sensitivity, we cannot understand their language. Thus, by doing the following practices, not only we receive the cosmic energy to enhance your vitality but also the cosmic bodies provide us with a guiding force in our lives which gives us mental strength.

Preparatory exercises of Japa

Japa or *svādhyāya* is done by silently repeating a mantra or another sound (Part II, 44) in order to silence the activities of the mind. If *japa* is addressed to some particular energy, deity or power, there is oneness of the adept with that particular object one is aiming at. Let me give you the method of *japa* by the repetition of the smallest mantra OṂ(ॐ). Its meaning, figurative form and significance have been already explained in Section II.

Sit down in a relaxed position, preferably cross-legged. Do some *prāṇāyāma* exercise and then start to repeat OṂ. You should synchronise the breathing with the recitation. Begin by repeating the word OṂ with each breath. Slowly increase the time of repetition by prolonging the sound AU... and ending with a prolonged nasal Ṃ... . Repeat several times without a break. During recitation, the eyes should be shut and the symbol of OṂ should be visualised at the point between your two eyes.

After the initial practice, begin to visualise the figurative form of OṂ in details and synchronise it with your recitation and breath. As you commence to chant, bring your thoughts to the upper part of the figure, which is like number 3. As you proceed with chanting AU... visualise the whole form except the half moon with a dot in it. This latter should be visualised when you come to the nasal Ṃ....

As you know from Sūtra 27, Part I, the repetition of mantra of the OṂ is called *praṇava.* When you reach an advanced state, you should repeat the mantra silently. You recite the mantra in your mind and visualise its form as described above.

If this practice is done persistently, it helps to enhance concentration and brings stillness of mind. Gradually, you will develop the ability to stop your thought process when you wish to or shut your mind from certain theme to come to another. But like the *yogāsanas* and *prāṇāyāma*, this also needs constant practice in order to gain success.

Japa: a part of your daily life

The basic importance of *japa* is to attain a thought-free mind and ability to direct the mind in the desired direction as and when one wants. Attaining a thought-free mind is a precondition for developing spiritual energy. Practice of *japa* should not be limited to a daily 10 minutes session but should become an integral part of your life. Despite the very busy schedules most people have, all of us still have plenty of free time that can be beneficially utilised for the practice of *japa*. For example, when we drive, wait for a train, bus or a visitor or wait to go inside a doctor's clinic or hundreds of other situations like that, we can use that time beneficially for practising *japa*. It keeps the mind fresh, enhances memory and gives calmness. It enhances the *sattva* element in us. You can do *japa* on sun, moon, stars, trees, flowers, stones, mountains etc. to receive the cosmic energy in abundance. Just look at the forms of the natural and beautiful objects around you and keep their image in your mind. Let the mind be still for few moments on that image. Most of the time, we keep thinking about people, problems, work etc. and pass by the natural splendour without drawing this energy within us. In fact, if we get into the habit of assimilating cosmic energy within us rather than wasting our energy by letting our mind, wander, the problems we are worried about will be solved with the wisdom from within us. In the next step, I will describe some very simple exercises for the intake of the cosmic energy. Your effort lies in remembering to do them and to incorporate them in your way of life in such a manner that they become a part of your daily life. You will realise that you live on a different plane of existence than you used to and this energy will bring you strength and wisdom.

Exercises for receiving the cosmic energy

These exercises involve looking with concentration at the natural sources of energy around you, shutting your eyes with the form of the object in your mind and taking a deep breath and holding your breath while concentrating on the form of the object. Then let the breath out while you have still the image of the object in your mind. It is like you are drinking the splendour, beauty and energy of the object. This process is not time consuming nor you need privacy or a special place for it. If you have the possibility, you may do the exercise with several breaths but make it a habit to do it at least with one breath.

Five fundamental elements in one form or the other are the source of tremendous energy and we can easily concentrate on them. I will describe below the symbolic significance of some cosmic sources of energy and you can take in the specific energy according to the time and need. When you practice this for a long time, you get an experience and can do the exercises in abstraction. That means that the object aimed at does not have to be present—you can concentrate on its form. For example, the sun is not there at night but you can keep its form and significance in mind and do the exercise.

Sun: The sun is the source of light, symbol of time and it is the cosmic fire, which is in the form of *pitta* within our bodies. Sun is also the symbol of brilliance, intellect, name and fame. Sun shows us the way, literally and otherwise in life. Therefore, for achievements and success in a particular field, you should draw constantly the energy from the sun. If you lose your way, do not lose your nerve; concentrate on the sun in the above-described method. The sun also symbolises activity and *rajas* and thus, the right side of the body. It represents the masculine energy in the body. If you are a shy person, subdued in your emotions and have difficulty to express yourself, assimilate regularly the sun's energy. In Part III, Sūtra 26, Patañjali says that the knowledge of the universe comes by performing *saṃyama* on the sun.

Moon: The moon represents the night, the *tamas*, the feminine aspect, and the left side of the body. The moon is the symbol of wisdom. It is cold by nature as opposited to the sun. If you get easily excited and angry, if you are hyperactive, assimilate moon's energy regularly.

Stars, open sky and the vast spaces: All these symbolise ether. It is the first of the five elements of our existence. Patañjali says that a divine power of hearing develops in the adept by performing *saṃyama* on ether. Assimilate the energy from the sources which signify ether in order to expand yourself at diverse levels of existence, to fulfil a wish to travel or achieve something which seems difficult and far reaching.

Air: The second of the five elements, which constitute us, is assimilated by us constantly in the form of *prāṇa* energy and its importance has already been told. One can perform *prāṇāyāma* with the concentration of the elemental form of air specially to gain courage, enthusiasm and to get over emotions like fear and insecurity.

Water: Like the sun, Water is everywhere around us. Many of you may live on the bank of a water source. Water does not flow itself but it represents the flow of life. It is because of its fluidity that the vitality essential for life is possible. Water is the greatest purifier and is used in many ways for spiritual therapy. Many problems in life are caused due to our rigid behaviour or rigidity in another way. You should constantly assimilate energy from lakes, rivers, seas, falling rain, moving clouds and other sources of water you come across. You may wish that with the energy of water, our minds and bodies might stay pure.

Earth: Earth is the giver, it protects us, it shelters us and it nourishes us. It is symbolic of stability, tolerance and procreation. You can assimilate its energy in many forms— from trees, flowers, crystals, rocks, mountains etc. Along with water, earth makes the solid structure of our body. Therefore, you should assimilate its energy for healing wounds and for healing other ailments where an active regeneration is required. Learn stability and tolerance from this energy and use it also for fulfilling a wish for fertility. Assimilate from this energy the creative power and modesty.

Knowledge about the bodily systems

In Part III, Sūtra 29, Patañjali has said that the knowledge about the bodily systems is obtained by performing *saṃyama* on the navel circle. This knowledge is very important for us in the context of Āyurvedic yoga. However, to learn *saṃyama* is a difficult thing for ordinary human beings and it requires tremendous practice, time and effort. I have made a simple version with *prāṇāyāma* and mental concentration on a single object, which will serve the purpose of self-diagnosis.

Sit down cross-legged or in another sitting posture if you have mastered one. First do some exercises of *prāṇāyāma* and then try to obtain a thought-free mental state with *japa.* Imagine the form of the syllable OṂ on your navel and go on doing *japa.* When your mind is fully concentrated, do only the silent repetition of the mantra. The next step is to send the *prāṇa* energy to your navel and to keep it there for as long as you can. Smoothly exhale and then hold the lungs without air. Your mind and thought process should stay still and you should have only the image of your navel region. To attain the single-pointedness, you will require repeated and persistent practice. This state of concentration should be prolonged and the respiration will be subdued when you have attained a continuous state of concentration. The energy circles radiating from the navel point will surround you. If your humours are in equilibrium, these circles are quite still. If you have *vāta* in imbalance, you may have difficulty in prolonging the state of concentration. If you are nervous or hectic and are anxious about something, you may see vibrations in the energy circles. When the energy circles are greyish and at times they are disappearing, that also speaks for *vāta* vitiation.

Red, orange and blue energy circles are indicative of *pitta* imbalance. If these colours are too strong, it is the vitiation of this humour. White, thick and viscous lines around you indicate *kapha* imbalance. It may be a thick circle instead of lines in case of the vitiation of this humour. Thus, with this method, you can visualise the state of your bodily humours. After the diagnosis, you should take appropriate measures to establish the equilibrium of the humours. Continue this practice and you will see that with your treatment, your energy envelop alters.

It is possible that you may have altering situation in your energy circle. There may be indications of the imbalance of the two humours at a time. If you are unable to observe circles in the energy envelope and there is a confusion of lines and colours, that is indicative of complete imbalance and you are in need of proper cure from a physician.

This practice can also be used for healing a particular body part. When you have formed the energy envelope, bring your attention on the affected part. The idea is to harmonise the affected part with the rest and it is done by supplying the energy from the navel circle.

Knowledge about the state of mind

The three states of mind are *sattva, rajas* and *tamas.* The knowledge about them is obtained by concentrating on the plexus, also known as the solar plexus. In Āyurveda, this area is known as *hṛdaya. Hṛdaya* is very important as it is considered to be the site of the soul. From Āyurvedic point of view, this part is the most vital in the whole body. The literal meaning of the word *hṛdaya* is heart but this term in Āyurvedic anatomy also signifies the part of the body containing the three most vital organs—heart, lungs and liver.

Begin to concentrate on plexus with some symbolic form like OṂ or the sun. Do this concentration exercise twice a day. Send *prāṇa* energy to this region constantly during the concentration sessions or otherwise. Remember that this is the most vital region of your body, the domain of soul and has the greatest concentration of the *prāṇic* energy. After a constant practice, you will be able to locate the exact point of the concentric energy. When you have uninterrupted concentration at this point, you may face some hurdles. The accumulative *tamas* will come out of your mind in the process of purifications. You may face fearfulness, sweating, trembling etc. With a constant practice, these are gradually thrown out and your mind is purified. You reach the domain of *sattva* where there is only purity and light. If you wish to heal certain part of your body, concentrate first on that part and then simply do your concentration session on the plexus as described above. The details of the healing techniques will be described in my forthcoming book on Spiritual Healing.

Note: The above-described energy envelopes around us, in both the cases are described as different states of aura by some. In fact, in all human beings, we do see the state of the three qualities of the mind if we ourselves have sattva domination. The proportion of the three guṇas makes us look different at different times. The same human being emits different kinds of energy when he/she is angry or getting up after a concentration session. Most of us see that but do not know how to explain this difference and try to justify it. We try to impose it on outward factors like weather, clothes etc.

Marmas and the subtle body

My research work always involved operating upon animals as I was studying the degeneration and regeneration of the neuro-muscular junctions. From my understanding, I always operated in the similar manner and with the same skill, but at times, either the animal bled to death or just died after several hours or few days of the operation. I thought that this might happen due to the difference in the energy levels or resistance of the individual animals. Years later, when I studied *Suśruta Saṃhitā*[9] in detail, I realised why certain animals died during or after I had operated upon them. During the operations, I was hurting at their *marma* points. These are the vital points of the body which are very sensitive to any shock or injury. According to Suśruta, "*Marmas* are those points where muscles, blood vessels, nerves, bones and ligaments combine together. These points have also the *prāṇa* in more concentration. If these points are, in one way or the other attacked, the functions of the sense organs such as speech, tactile sensation, taste, sight etc. are disturbed. The mental state also gets deranged and symptoms like forgetfulness, regret, depression and falling down etc. begin to appear."[10] Total number of *marmas* in the body is 107. The arms and legs have 11 each, the thorax and abdomen have 12 *marmas*, back has 14 and neck and head have 37 *marmas.*[11] Suśruta further adds that *marmas* have a concentration of air, fire and water elements, *rajas, tamas* and *sattva,* and the concentration of the energy from the soul and that is the reason why upon being hurt on these points, one does not live any more.[12]

Suśruta was a great surgeon of all times and his thorough and systematic study of the *marmas* was for the purpose of surgery. The surgeon should have a very precise understanding of these points and be extremely carefull not to hurt them during surgery. The knowledge of the *marmas* existed in India before the physicians

---

9 Suśruta was a great physician and surgeon of the 6th century BC, which is also considered to be the golden age of Āyurveda. His treatise is known as *Suśruta Saṃhitā. Caraka Saṃhitā* by *Caraka,* which is referred to throughout this book and *Suśruta Saṃhitā* are the two principal treatises of Āyurveda from that period. Patañjali wrote the *Yogasūtra* nearly during the same period.

10 *Suśruta Saṃhitā, Śarīrasthānam,* VI, 15.

11 *Ibid* VI, 5.

12 *Ibid* VI, 35

systematised it and used it in surgery. Earlier this wisdom was used for self-protection, in martial arts and during wars.

For a person with reductionist approach to science and medicine and with purely materialistic basis, it is difficult to understand *marmas.* However, I want to remind you that *marmas* are something anatomical and with practice and experience they can be seen. But the concept with *prāṇic* energy and vitality and that even the area around them should be fully protected,[13] may not be understandable to those who look at reality in a very limited sensuous terms. *Marmas* are not exactly the energy points of the subtle body but are anatomically located quite close to them. You must remember that the subtle body and its energy points do not require physical space. Besides, I have already explained above that the *prāṇa* energy is the linking factor of the part of the energy of the soul, which we have in each and every cell of the body. Thus, it is quite logical to think that if *marmas* are the special vital points of the body and specifically have more *prāṇa* energy as well as the elements air, fire and water, they cannot be too far from the subtle energy points. The cosmic reality has different levels. There is the concrete and material level that can be perceived with the senses. Then there is a subtle level that is felt in many different ways but not perceived or technically measured and so on. There is a level that falls between these two categories—it is the transition from the sensuous to the subtle. Or it is the combination of the sensuous and subtle. That is where I would place *marmas.*

The idea of this brief discription of the *marmas* is to make you realise the different aspects of the 'living' in the body. Our purpose in Āyurvedic yoga is not to let this vital part subside, rather we should make every effort to revitalise and rejuvenate it.

In the context of *marma,* I want to take up a theme upon which I am often questioned in Germany and my opinion was sought. Many of my students have studied yoga with a group that teaches you to concentrate on the different *marmas* for various cures and to release stress and tension. I certainly agree that bringing the intentness of the mind on specific *marmas* will bring positive and beneficial results. As it is clear from the above discussion, *marmas*

---

13 *Suśruta Saṃhitā Śarīrasthānam,* VI, 41.

have concentration of the vital energy, force or *prāṇa* and it is quite obvious that this force which interconnects and makes the body a unity and links it with the cosmos will harmonise the 'living element' within us. Thus, I completely agree with the application of yogic concentration methods on the *marmas* in our body for the purpose of cure and healing and to revitalise our forces. As cited above, Suśruta says that any kind of physical attack on the *marmas* will effect our sensuous faculty and will diminish our sensuous power. In this light, it is quite obvious that protecting and concentrating on *marmas* and supplying them with *prāṇic* energy will enhance the sensuous faculties. But we should keep in mind that the results obtained will not be the same as by concentrating on the major subtle energy points described above. These results are at a higher spiritual level. The two techniques described above with the navel and the plexus help us to scan and visualise our body and mind by reaching the spiritual level. We have talked about the spiritual level throughout this book. When the mind becomes thought-free, it attains oneness with the soul rather than with the sensuous physical body and we 'see' another dimension of reality at this level. Concentrating on the *marmas* may provide us a stepping stone from the physical to the spiritual.

Protecting the 'living' inside you from attacks

We are constantly attacked by outer forces and we should learn to protect ourselves from these in order to keep our vital elements intact at diverse levels of our existence. Throughout this part of the book, I have mentioned so many of these factors like hectic pace of life, stress, tension, *tamas* thoughts and so on. I have given the methods to save oneself from the negative thoughts as well as to deal with tension etc. You must always remember that a disease or an ailment does not come to us instantaneously. Very gradually, the 'living element' in us is wounded, partly dies and the rest of the 'living element' struggles to keep the whole system of the being in order. But it is not complete, it is partial and finally it fails to maintain an order- and we have a major disorder. Half of my adult life I have done research on how to cure disorders and finally reached the conclusion that we should prevent disorders because when they are there, most of the time it is not possible to cure them and if possible, then only partially. Several years ago, I had some problems in my left knee. It was mainly caused by my over-enthusiasm for our Āyurvedic garden in the Himalayan mountains for which I wanted to do the plantation myself. My urbanised body could not take so much physical stress and the knee ligament gave way. Obviously, there were some inner factors adding to it, which brought this disorder. Despite so much persistence from the family and friends, I did not go to the specialist physicians in Europe and let the knee heal by itself aided by some rational and spiritual therapy. However, upon my return to India, I went to see a very well known Āyurvedic physician in Delhi. After inquiring about the problem, Triguna ji commented, "Thank God you resisted the forces and did not get your knee operated because an organ is never the same after the operation." Well, this was the matter of external intervention. But internally, when a disorder occurs in the system at a bigger scale, it is never possible to bring it back to the original vitality and force. Therefore, my repeated message is—SAVE YOURSELF! Simple methods of Āyurvedic yoga will enlighten your path in this direction. The eternal wisdom of yoga and Āyurveda, which is not time or space bound, will help save the humanity from ailments. Let us pay homage to the ancient sages-, the exponents of this wisdom.

OṂ SHANTI

DR. VERMA'S CENTERS IN INDIA

This book on Ayurveda is meant to be a very simple guide so that you can use Ayurvedic practices in your daily life. I encourage you to change your life by taking small steps—exercise you can do at home, remedies you can make at home, the 16-minute program, and so on. The herbs and spices introduced here are easily available. They belong to traditional Indian and Pakistani cuisine. I have tried to provide the Hindi names along with the English and Latin names for herbs and spices so you can locate them in Indian food stores.

Ayurveda is a complete holistic system of living and deals with all aspects of life. I am well aware that it is not easy to switch from a fragmented approach to a holistic one—either philosophically or in the various practical aspects of life. Therefore, I travel in Europe to give lectures, seminars and weekend workshops on "Ayurveda a Way of Life" and other subjects, such as holistic sexuality, Ayurvedic nutrition, stress management with yoga and Ayurveda, and so on. These can be organized by invitation and I am always in Europe between August and November of every year. I am happy to travel to the United States to lecture as well. For providing practical training, we have two centers in India, one in Noida (a suburb of New Delhi) and the other in the Himalayan mountains, 400 kilometers north of New Delhi, on the bank of the Ganga. There are short term — one to three week intensive programs — meant to provide you with a living experience of Ayurveda so that you can continue for the rest of your lives with saptakarma, Ayurvedic cooking, spiritual living, and so on.

The main purpose of this network is to spread the message of health care in the world and to bring about a health revolution. I want to make you aware that you are responsible for your own health and you should live your life with the totality of being. The first priority of life is to safeguard your existence. It is not about just staying alive, it's about your quality of life and living with a happy disposition (prasanchitta).

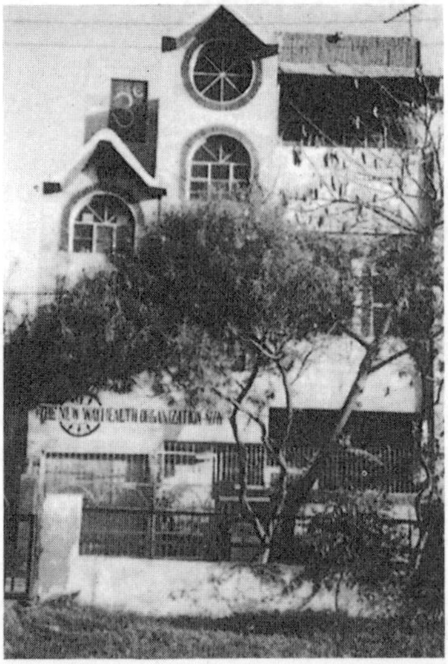

Figure 50. ***The Noida Center near New Delhi***

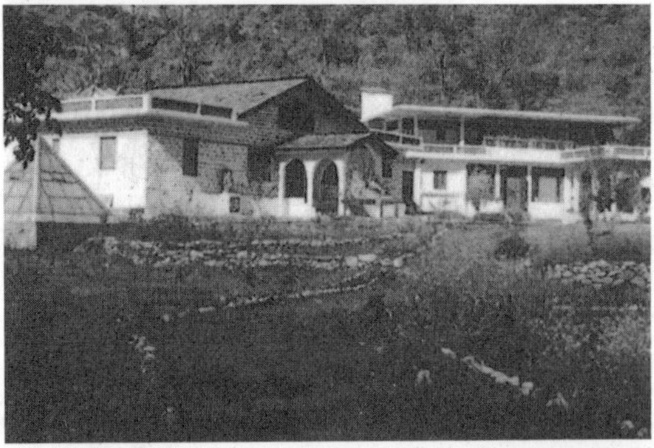

Figure 51. ***The Himalayan Center***

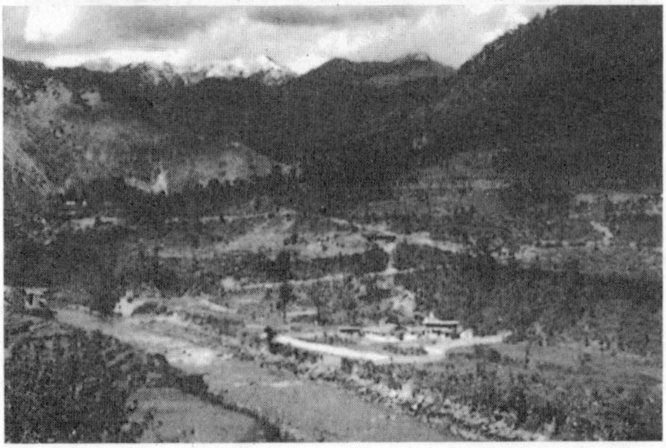

Figure 52. ***The View from the Himalayan center will totally change your outlook of life***

I hope you will benefit from this ancient Ayurvedic wisdom and that you will help to spread the Ayurvedic message of holistic living and join me in this crusade for health.

Dr. Vinod Verma
The New Way Health Organization .NOW.
A-130, Sector 26, Noida 201301, UP, India
Telephone 091-11-852 7820; Fax 091-11-855-2368

ABOUT THE AUTHOR

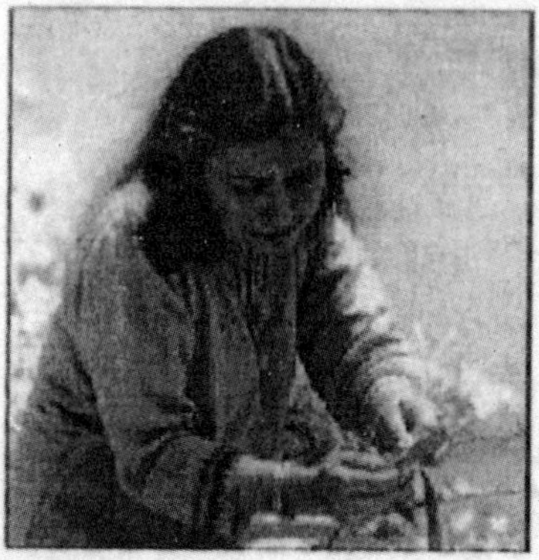

Dr. Vinod Verma assimilated yoga and Ayurveda from her father and grandmother. She earned a Ph.D. in Reproduction Biology from Panjab University, Chandigarh and a Ph.D. in Neurobiology from the University of Paris (old Sorbonne). She got her training in Neurobiology from the prestigious National Institutes of Health, Bethesda, USA, and worked at the Max Planck Institute in Freiburg, Germany.

At the peak of career with a pharmaceutical company in Germany, Dr. Verma realised that the modern Western approach to health is fragmented, illogical and uni-dimensional (non-holistic). The mental and spiritual aspects are lacking and all our resources are put in curing diseases rather than trying to stay healthy. She returned to her traditional past, studied Patanjali and other texts on yoga and learnt the scriptural tradition of Ayurveda from her Ayurvedic guru, Acharya Priya Vrat Sharma.

A Scientific Exposition of Patanjali's Yogasutras was her first book that she began writing in 1986 and after years of research, this book was published in 1996. She has written seven more books on yoga, Ayurveda and women's health and these books are published in different languages of the world.

Dr. Verma founded The New Way Health Organisation in 1986 to spread the message of holistic health care and spiritual living. She is totally dedicated to revive the spiritual tradition of yoga and integrate it with Ayurveda for health and healing. She hosts seminars, lectures and workshops and has been interviewed on TV and radio programmes all over the world. She has made a film on Ayurveda in collaboration with German television and this film has been shown in 130 languages in 100 different countries. She has also numerous scientific papers published in international journals.